BUGGIES, BLIZZARDS, AND BABIES

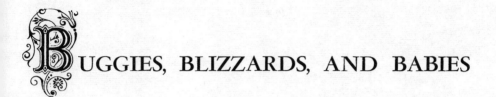

BUGGIES, BLIZZARDS, AND BABIES

CORA FREAR HAWKINS

The Iowa State University Press, Ames

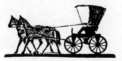

CORA FREAR HAWKINS is a native Iowan, born in the small town of Sloan and educated at Morningside College in nearby Sioux City, from where she was graduated in 1907.

The experiences recounted here reveal a life influenced by warm childhood memories of her father, a country doctor in active practice for many years, beginning in 1882. As a child Cora accompanied him whenever possible.

Studying by kerosene lamp, usually in a kitchen warmed by a corncob fire, she finished high school at sixteen and entered college. There she met Lon A. Hawkins. After their marriage in 1908, they made their home in Washington, D.C., for thirty-four years. On her husband's retirement from the U.S. Department of Agriculture in 1942 they bought a fruit farm near Eugene, Oregon, where Mrs. Hawkins still lives.

Mrs. Hawkins, a member of the National League of American Pen Women, is active in writers' groups and church work. Although this is her first book, she has published features, stories, short articles, and poems.

© 1971 The Iowa State University Press
Ames, Iowa 50010. All rights reserved
Composed and printed by The Iowa State University Press
First edition, 1971
International Standard Book Number: 0–8138–0395–0
Library of Congress Catalog Card Number: 74–137091

TO MY GRANDCHILDREN in the hope that through this book they may know something of the character and the rugged way of life of their great-grandparents, Edwin and Sue Frear.

CONTENTS

Preface   ix

1 / The Blizzard   3

2 / Homely Beginnings   9

3 / A Goal Attained   16

4 / The First Hundred Days Were the Hardest   25

5 / A Doctor's Wife in the Nineties   31

6 / The Doctor's Children   49

7 / Horse and Buggy Doctor   62

8 / A-Calling We Would Go   72

9 / Down in the Bend   87

10 / Office Assistant in Pigtails   95

11 / The New House   104

12 / Quarantine in the Nineties   111

13 / School Days   120

14 / Babies—Ten Dollars Delivered   132

15 / Transition   145

16 / Grandfather Frear   154

17 / A Son, to Become a Doctor   164

18 / Adjustment   173

19 / And One Clear Call   183

PREFACE

W HEN at the age of seventy-three my father suffered a stroke, I went from my home in Washington, D.C., to stay with him in the Sioux City hospital. A nurse took care of his physical needs, leaving me free to talk with his visitors. There were many from all walks of life, from three to eighty-three years old, but they had one thing in common—each one wanted to tell me of some kindness aside from his professional services that Father had done for them. Their stories, their affection, moved me so deeply that I felt it must all be written down. On the Pullman on the way home I asked for a table and began writing. So it was that the last chapter of *Buggies, Blizzards, and Babies* was written first.

Over the years other incidents came to mind or were told to me. Under the direction of Professor Sylvan N. Karchmer of the University of Oregon, I began shaping them into a book. I had encouragement and constructive criticism from fellow members of our Eugene Branch, National League of American Pen Women.

I had spent so much time with my father on rides into the country as a child and later working with him in the office, that memory has played a large part in the writing of this book. But while I have had to fill in, add dialogue, and for obvious reasons often change names, locale, and other details, every incident related is based on an actual experience of my father or one of the family.

I had access to a great many old letters and to a diary which Father kept as a young man, and on visits to his old home in Pennsylvania I learned much about his background and early life.

I have checked medical books and biographies of early phy-

ix

sicians for the history and development of medical practice; an important source of such information has been *The Doctors Mayo,* by Helen Clapesattle. Dr. Will Mayo began his studies at the University of Michigan in September 1880, the month before Father registered at the Medical School of the State University of Iowa, so the Mayo records were very helpful.

For checking names, dates, and incidents in the early history of the area in which Father practiced, I was fortunate in having three small books: *The History of Salix,* two volumes, and *Sloan, Yesterday and Today,* all compiled and printed by Louis N. Duchaine of Sloan.

To the above and to all who have helped and encouraged me in producing this book, I. am deeply grateful.

BUGGIES, BLIZZARDS, AND BABIES

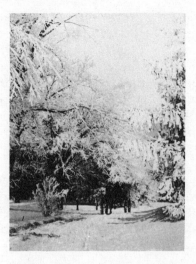

Snow had fallen, snow on snow,
Snow on snow,
In the bleak mid-winter,
Long ago.
—ROSSETTI, *Mid-Winter*

Chapter *1*

THE BLIZZARD

S ue Frear, dozing in a rocker by the kitchen stove, was aroused by the sound of the wind whistling around the chimney. She drew her gray shawl more closely about her shoulders and went to the window. Cupping her hands, she shaded her eyes against the reflection of lamplight on the glass, but try as she might she could see no light other than her own in the little Iowa village.

It was late. Sue looked hopefully for some sign that the snowstorm was subsiding, but it seemed rather to be increasing in fury as the wind whirled clouds of fine snowflakes past the house and down the dark street. She strained to see further, but she could see only her own shadow quivering in the patch of light on

3

the shifting snow and the dim outline of the house across the street where drifts were piling halfway to the eaves.

But Sue's thoughts were less on her neighbors in the town than on a farmhouse ten miles away, nestled in the edge of the hills, where a young mother fought for her life and that of her unborn child. And somewhere on the bleak prairie that lay between, its once lush grasses now buried under a heavy white blanket, Sue's doctor husband, Edwin, battled the stinging cold and wind in the darkness, trying to reach the young wife before it was too late.

Earlier in the evening just as they were finishing supper, a young man on horseback had pulled up. The doctor ran out carrying a blanket to throw over the horse and helped the rider down and into the house. As he took the man's coat and gently massaged his numb hands, he asked, "What brings you out in such a storm?"

Speaking with difficulty through half-frozen lips, the visitor said, "Lige Adams sent me. His wife's having a baby and they need help."

He declined Sue's offer to fix him some supper, but he drank a cup of hot coffee eagerly. She refilled his cup and he continued, "There's a neighbor woman with her now. She's a right good hand with baby cases too, but this one ain't comin' right. Breech case, she called it, and she don't know how to turn it. Said they'd have to send for you. And please hurry, Doc! That poor woman's been in labor since some time in the night, and when I left it didn't look like she'd hold out much longer."

Then, answering the doctor's questions, he gave a grim picture of the weather and driving conditions across the sparsely settled country. After three days of blizzard, the roads and even the fence-posts were completely covered, while the powderlike snow filled the air, making the few trees and the windmills invisible.

"Of course, it was still daylight when I started out, and I could keep some sense of direction," he said. "It was pretty dark by the time I hit the prairie, but do you know, that darned horse seemed to know I was headed for Sloan, so I just let him take over. I'd hate to try to go back now. Lige told me to go to the hotel and stay 'til it clears off. I'd better get on over there now." He got up, rubbed his hands together over the stove, pulled on his heavy coat and gloves, and said, "Thanks for the coffee, Mrs.

4

Frear. That sure hit the spot. And good luck to you, Doc," and he went out into the storm.

Before the door had closed, Sue saw with a feeling of helplessness that the doctor was already preparing for the trip. She did not try to dissuade him—she knew it would be useless. Then too she had a bond of sympathy with the young mother, because her own baby, their second, was due in a few weeks; so she went about quietly helping her husband get ready. Bricks were always kept warming on the back of the stove; now she pulled them over the fire, started a fresh pot of coffee, and spread the heavy wolfskin coat and fur robe over the backs of chairs to warm in front of the oven.

The doctor changed to heavier clothing, with the added protection of a pair of chamois-skin drawers under his trousers; then he went to the barn, harnessed the team, hitched them to the sleigh, and drove to the door. The horses stomped and jingled the sleigh bells, while inside he warmed his hands and made final preparations.

All this time, two-year-old Edna sat in her high chair beside the table, her rag doll held tight in her plump arms. Edna was seldom quiet for long, but tonight while the young man was there her wide eyes had kept looking from one parent to the other as if disturbed by the tension in the air, until her head dropped forward and, pillowed by the rag doll on the tray of her chair, she fell asleep. Now she roused up and held out her hands to her father. He picked her up and swung her to the ceiling, so that she laughed and begged, "More! More!"

But he kissed her and put her down, saying, "More tomorrow, Baby! You be a good girl now and take care of your mother."

Sue clung to him as he held her for a moment and kissed her tenderly, then she helped him into his fur coat; he pulled on fur-lined gloves and cap, picked up his robes, the medicine case, and the all-important brown leather satchel, and went out to the sleigh. Sue followed with a jug of hot coffee and the hot bricks, putting one on the floor and one on each side of him to keep his hands warm; she helped pull the robes up around him and tuck them in, then hurried back into the house and watched silently from the window as long as she could see the sleigh, fully aware that the chances were against his finding his way in the storm, realizing that if he became lost his survival would be most difficult.

She tried to put it all out of her mind, for Edna was tugging

5

at her skirt. Though tempted to keep the child up for company, she carried her to the rocker and undressed her, then played games with the pink toes. Edna laughed aloud until her eyelids began to droop, then Sue carried her to the bedroom, trying to remain cheerful as she kissed her and tucked her in bed.

Back in the kitchen, Sue looked at the clock and tried to determine how far the doctor had gone, and decided that he was about to start across the prairie. She sat down at the table and buried her head in her arms and prayed for his safety.

The stillness of the room, broken only by the steady ticking of the clock inside and the howling wind outside, depressed her. She got up to clear the table, glad for the noisy clatter of the dishes, and prolonged the task as long as possible. As she wiped the last dish and hung up her dishpan, certain comforting verses from the Psalm the doctor had read that morning came to mind: "Thou shalt not be afraid for the terror by night. . . . For He shall give His angels charge over thee." She said them over as she pulled the rocker close to the stove and sat down. Her eyes were heavy, but to go to bed was unthinkable.

Now she leaned wearily against the window frame, found the wind had changed, and fine snow was drifting in around the sash. She shivered, but in spite of the cold she continued to watch the storm until she thought of her unborn child, and remembered that much depended on her keeping well. She pulled down the shade to keep out some of the cold, but that made her feel more alone and she raised it again. She went to fill the stove with wood, then returned to the window, and presently she realized that she was pacing back and forth across the room.

The clock began to strike the hour and Sue paused to count the strokes, although she knew it was midnight. Then she went to see that Edna was well covered, for the bedroom was cold, there being no heat except what came in during the day from the kitchen and sitting-room stoves.

The light from the kitchen gave a warm glow as she tiptoed toward the bed. The crib was comfortable, she thought with pride. Many people used trundle beds, built on low casters so they could be rolled under the big beds when not in use, but Sue disapproved of them because they were exposed to the cold drafts and dust of the floor.

Together she and the doctor had planned and made this bed, large enough for two children. Its board sides were painted light

6

gray; the wooden slats were close together; the corn-shuck tick was soft and springy, for Sue had split the husks to give them extra elasticity and had carefully removed all the cob-butts. The quilt was made from pieces of the doctor's old wool suits, discarded when they could no longer be patched. Surely Edna was as warm and cozy as loving hands could make her.

It comforted Sue just to look at the little girl, whose round pink face, even in repose, appeared ready to wrinkle up any moment and break into mischievous laughter. Surely no harm would come to the little family while Edna was so secure in her charmed world. Tomorrow she would run about and get into mischief as usual. She would crawl under the breakfast table and pinch her father's legs, then run before he could catch her, backing into the farthest corner with her hands braced against the wall, and laugh until her short braids bobbed up and down. And the doctor, nearly bursting with pride and affection, would say under his breath, "Dog-gone it, why couldn't you have been a boy?"

A boy! A son to go on trips with him, to help in the office; later to study medicine and work into his practice! That was the doctor's dream. He was building a practice that he could be proud of, and Sue shared both his ambition and his wish for a son.

Maybe they would have a boy this time—they would soon know. Then again like a stab of pain came the fear that she had been fighting. What if her doctor husband were not there when her baby was born? She laid her cheek against the little girl's hair for reassurance and kissed her gently, tucked a chubby fist under the cover, and with a last loving look as she closed the door, she went back to the kitchen.

Looking about for something to do, she brought wood from the lean-to and nearly froze her hands as she did so, then made a pot of coffee and set it on the back of the stove. Again she paced the floor, glancing often at the clock, and always the prayer was on her lips, "Father, bring him back to me!"

At last, tired and cold, she again sat down in the rocking chair by the stove and pulled a blanket around her. From here she could look through the window and watch for the first signs of daylight. The clock struck three. Surely if the doctor were to reach his patient at all, he had arrived by now and had accomplished his errand. It was good to remember that once he started home, the instinct of the horses would be a safe guide for the re-

7

turn trip; now she forced herself to think of him as being homeward bound.

Suddenly startled, Sue realized that she had been asleep, for through the window she saw early dawn lighting the eastern sky. It had stopped snowing and the wind had gone down. She hurried to build up the fire, then stopped to listen. It *was* sleigh bells! Down the street came the welcome sound, then the sleigh turned into the lane beside the house and she heard her husband's voice: "Hullo! Sue? Oh, Sue! I'm home!"

She threw the door wide open and he stumbled from the sleigh up the steps and into her arms. Inside, he discarded the heavy gloves and coat for lighter ones. He took only a swallow of the coffee she offered. "I've got to take care of the horses," he said hoarsely as he started for the door.

She stopped him with her hand on his arm. "Tell me, were you in time?"

"I made it in time, with God's help," he said humbly. "They have a baby boy and everyone's fine."

She turned away, overcome with joy and relief. Her husband had risked his life that another might live, but he had come back to her.

And he was with her on that early March morning six weeks later when her baby was born. Again a blizzard was raging outside, but her husband was cheerful and confident, and she felt warm and unafraid. Presently she heard him say, "Well, Sue, we have another little girl." Later he brought the baby to the bedside. She looked at the little bald head and the puckered red face, smiled happily, and curved her arm to make a nest for her child.

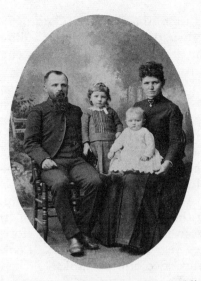

Dr. and Mrs. E. D. Frear were established
members of the Sloan community when they
posed in 1888 with daughters Edna and Cora.

Chapter 2

HOMELY BEGINNINGS

ORE THAN four years had passed since my red-faced
debut during the March blizzard, an event followed in
less than two years by the birth of my brother—the boy
who was to become the second Doctor Frear. My parents named
him Charles, a family name, but called him Charley. He was
toddling around now, a lovable little fellow, but frail, hence
always under Mother's watchful eye. Father proudly introduced
him as "my future partner," adding, "Someday my shingle will
read DRS. FREAR *AND* FREAR."

My sister Edna, now almost seven, was full of fun and mischief. Though blessed with a lot of common sense that made
most of her pranks harmless, she still kept Mother on the alert.
Since Edna and Charley, each for a different reason, demanded

9

much of Mother's time, that left me (Cora or Carrie—I answered to either) to my own devices. I usually followed Papa around when he was home and whenever possible went with him on his trips into the country.

Often in the morning, when the cheerful sound of the coffee mill told me that Mamma was up, I'd slip downstairs and climb into bed with Papa. He was never too tired to reach out an arm to pillow my head and cuddle me close, and we'd both sleep until called for breakfast.

On this warm day in midsummer we stood at the kitchen window, three blue-eyed towheads watching for Papa to come home for dinner. We looked across a vacant lot, lush with uncut prairie grasses, to the small business shops in the block beyond. Edna saw him first as he passed the grocery store, and, with an intuition beyond her years, she exclaimed, "Look, Mamma! I bet he's got some money. See how he walks?"

Mother laughed as she looked. "Sure enough! I guess someone has paid his bill," she said. Father strutted down the street, erect, head up, his usual short, quick steps now striking a buoyant note. His fingers were spread wide, his hands thrown out as he walked.

Little Charley and I were off on a run. We met him at the corner of the vacant lot. We reached up two small hands, each to grasp a forefinger held out to us. I chattered as we trotted along, while Charley echoed the words he could pronounce. I told him Mamma was making me a new dress and Edna fell and skinned her knee and a yellow kitty had come to our house and wouldn't go away and—when I paused for breath he said, "That's fine. I'm glad you were a good girl." He hadn't heard a word I said but as always he encouraged our conversation.

Now we were at the kitchen door. Mother, laughing, met us, her open hands held out to Father. "Give it to me!" she demanded. He stopped and looked at her, apparently surprised.

"Give you what?" he asked.

"Give me that money. Somebody paid you and I want it."

"Oh, go on!" he said, laughing back at her. "You're dreaming. Nobody ever pays a doctor."

The coffeepot sputtered over on the hot stove, and she turned to push it back. He slipped past her and dropped a handful of silver dollars on the table as he went to hang up his hat. She scooped the money into her apron pocket and said, "Oh, thank you, kind sir! That'll be a sack of flour, a slab of bacon, and shoes for the baby. Who paid you?"

"Chris Dahl. He sold a calf. How did you know?"

"A little bird told me."

"I'm going to shoot that bird," he said over the tin wash basin, as he splashed cold water on his face. "Someday he'll tell too much," he mumbled through the roller towel. Standing before the small looking glass he combed his dark, stubborn hair, then drew the metal backed comb through his black beard and stroked it thoughtfully. It wasn't a very heavy beard, nor long, according to nineteenth century standards, still it did add some dignity, and that was good since he was only about five feet seven inches tall, and boyishly slender.

His feet and hands were small; he used to say he never could have specialized in surgery, even had he cared for that field, because his fingers were too short. He had a round face with a sensitive mouth, and his grey eyes twinkled; he enjoyed a joke whether it was on himself or another.

He turned from the mirror and watched the final preparations for dinner. One thing was sure—he had chosen the right wife for a country doctor. Sue was interested in his work and accepted without complaint the sacrifices and economies necessary for her to make.

Father seemed to care nothing for money in itself. When he had it, he was generous with his family and was always ready to help a less fortunate friend. But when bills came due—a large part of them for office equipment and books—when old man Smith hounded him for the eight dollars monthly rent for the house, when a payment was demanded on a note he had once signed with an unscrupulous friend, or when pressures mounted and money was not forthcoming, then he looked worried, even angry, and walked with clenched fists held close to his sides, his depression complete and ill concealed. He was, of course, totally unaware of this transparency and probably wondered, as he watched his wife, how she had known he had money.

Now she looked up. "We can eat now if you are ready, Doctor." She had known him first as "Doctor," and called him this all through the years, never using his given name, Edwin, nor even the more familiar Ed.

"I'm ready," he answered, "and if it tastes as good as it smells, I'm willing."

He lifted Charley into his high chair while she filled a tureen from the black iron kettle and carried it steaming to the table. The teakettle sang cheerily; the geranium blooming on the windowsill picked up the green of the painted wainscoting and the red of the checkered tablecloth. Father said grace, then tucked his napkin in his vest and served generous helpings to each of us before filling his own plate.

"Gosh, that's good," he said, smacking his lips. It was his favorite meal, a New England boiled dinner. "I suppose this beef is some of what Anderson brought in on account. But these vegetables, they came from our own garden, didn't they?"

"Every one of them. Carrots, cabbage, onions, and all the rest," Mamma said. She laughed as she poured a glass of milk for each of us children. "And fresh milk from the cow." Later she handed him a piece of pie and said, "Lard in the crust from the Shipe account, apples from Ole West."

"That's good pie, too," he said as he finished his piece and shoved back his chair. "But there's nothing better than home-grown vegetables. I don't know which I enjoy most—raising them or eating them."

Father was an enthusiastic gardener, but he entertained no such feeling for milking the cow. He did that when necessary, but seemingly with a feeling of injured pride bred in his home state of Pennsylvania where, he told us, a man caught doing the milking was in disgrace.

He often talked about things "back east," and we always listened wide-eyed, almost unbelieving. Why, there were springs of good drinking water that came up right out of the ground! And you could catch trout in the creek just below the house; and in the millrace beside the shop, you could trap eels—long slippery fish that looked like snakes but were good to eat. Lots of berries grew wild, and there were trees everywhere. To children raised in a prairie town, in a township without even a small creek or pond, all this was like fairyland.

But we liked best to hear about the frogs that leaped and splashed in the millpond, then sat on the bank and held choir practice. Breathless, we would listen while he told us how an old bullfrog would puff out his throat till it looked like a balloon, then give a loud "PEEP!" From the other side of the pond would come an answering peep, then another and another, until dozens joined in the chorus. To hear Papa tell it, this made lovely music.

And he would say, his eyes misty, "Someday I'm going back east in the spring, just to hear the peepfrogs once more."

He had told us that, if collections were good, we might go back east before long, and as we finished dinner this warm day, we begged him to tell us more about his old home. But he looked out through the kitchen door, beyond Mamma's border of nasturtiums and mignonette, to his well-kept rows of vegetables, and said, "Some other time. Right now I've got to hoe the potatoes."

He had hardly gotten started when a man drove up and called to him, "They want you right away to Lars Iverson's. The old man's heart is acting up." That was a doctor's life.

Collections must have been good for a while; however I suspect that a sizable check from Father's brother Dana and his wife Cora made possible the visit in August. It had been twelve years since he had left home and gone west to finish his education. During that time he had acquired a profession and a family. We all went with him.

Mother thought the occasion called for a high silk hat, and insisted on his wearing one in order to make the proper impression on his relatives and friends. Many times I've heard him laugh about it. He'd say, "When I arrived in the East I found that every cab driver, every confidence man, every Negro who could afford it was wearing a stovepipe hat like mine, but nary a doctor did I see so decked out. I lost no time in finding me a kady hat, and soon some junkman had a silk topper all his own."

Edna and I were not concerned with what kind of hat he wore, but we were thrilled when he took us for a long walk to show us some of the places he loved as a boy. We walked up the road to the place where it widened to make room for eight or ten rigs in front of the general store, which, with the blacksmith shop, church, and a few other buildings and homes, made up the town of Beaumont. Beyond the store the road curved off to the left, across a wooden bridge where we leaned over the rail and he pointed out the frog pond. The peepers were silent, of course, because mating season was long past. We passed the schoolhouse, and at the top of the hill on one side of the road was the Methodist church; on the other, the cemetery where many of Father's ancestors were buried.

Now he led us back down through the woods, following a

path softly carpeted with pine needles. We stopped to watch two deer that drank from the creek. Seeing us, the buck stepped protectingly in front of his mate. Motionless, they stared at us until a loose stone slipped and clattered down hitting against the rocks, when they bounded away to hide in the scrub pines under the brow of the hill.

As we came out into a clearing we could see below us a group of houses known as Freartown, because all were occupied by members or relatives of the family. Uncle Dana and Aunt Cora (for whom I was named) lived in the large white one, and we were staying with them. Nearby was the shop where generations of Frears had worked at cabinet making and related projects. Many of the tools they used were made by hand, while the lathe and circular saw were powered by a waterwheel outside.

We ended our long walk at the shop, where Grandfather was now turning out a pair of crutches for a neighbor who had broken his leg.

Grandfather and his eighteen-year-old son, Charley, lived in a cottage across the creek from the shop with his widowed daughter, Carrie Scovall (I'd been named for her too), and her own small son, Jim. The house was small but solidly built. The splint-bottomed chairs had been made by a Frear of an earlier generation for his bride; the spool bedsteads were hand turned, with strong ropes to hold a featherbed or straw-filled tick.

Grandfather's full name was William Doctor Frear, the unusual middle name having been given him because he was the seventh son (in a family of seventeen children) and as such he was destined by old wives' tales to become a doctor. That destiny was left for his son to fulfill, but, considering the time and the locale, Grandfather did have a fair education. He read widely and was especially interested in history; because of his broad acquaintance and good memory where local people and events were concerned, he was sometimes consulted by historians and genealogists; for them he often supplied a missing link in a chain of known events.

Known as Squire Frear because he was justice of the peace, Grandfather also served the community as undertaker. My father, while still in school, had helped with this work, and occasionally he served alone as undertaker.

The coffins were made in the shop, using the different woods that were available in the area, such as hickory, beech, chestnut, and cherry, often finished with a stain made from black walnuts. Daughter Carrie lined the coffins with a crinkly cotton material of eggshell color. It was a profitable family enterprise; for a complete funeral Grandfather received twenty dollars!

The coffins were made wide at the top, and narrowed nearly to a point at the foot. In his spare time Grandfather made lids and stored them for later use, so he had several on hand when a professional undertaker moved into the community and took over the business. A few coffin lids are still to be found in the homes of Grandfather's thrifty descendants. Padded, they make excellent ironing boards.

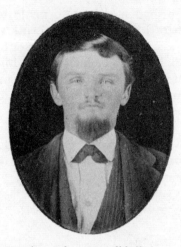

A mustache and goatee did little to disguise Edwin Frear's youthful looks as he began his medical studies January 1, 1876.

Chapter 3

A GOAL ATTAINED

PROBABLY Father's boyhood home as we saw it had changed little since Grandfather brought his bride, the former Elizabeth Parrish, to the community. Here all their six children were born; the oldest, my father, whom they named Edwin Daniel, arrived on May 3, 1854. Except for one little girl who died, they all grew up here; Father was the only one to make a permanent home more than a few miles away. Although I was only four at the time of our visit, I remembered many places and people, and visited there often after my marriage, when I lived in Washington, D.C.

Notable among the older relatives were Grandfather's sister Almira and Grandmother's sister Esther, known as Aunt Almi and Aunt Tet. They told me many things about Father's childhood.

Teenagers at the time he was born, they both lived into their nineties; they had seen three generations come and grow up in their own families, and still both insisted "little Ed" was the most wonderful baby of them all. For one thing, they said he seldom cried; if he fell down he would look surprised but say nothing, then get up, brush himself off, and go on with his play. They considered it prophetic of the way he would meet his problems in later life.

They laughed about an incident when he was five. They told him that Aunt Leafy Jackson, a midwife whom he feared and disliked, had brought him a sweet baby sister; he refused to look at her. Later they happened to look out the window just as Ed crossed the bridge that led to the main road. He struggled with a large bundle which he was holding defiantly when they caught up with him. "Don't like Aunt Leafy," he said. "Don't want her baby. I take it back." When they convinced him that it was Mamma's baby and that she loved it very much, he gave in and let them take the baby to its mother.

Probably what most impressed the aunts about my father was his love for school. There never was the problem of his playing hooky from school—quite the contrary. Even if he were sick and told to stay in bed, he would watch for a chance to slip out and run away to school. Aunt Almi remembered that when Ed was old enough to take his turn at the spring plowing, he worried because it would interfere with his school.

He talked it over with his younger brother, Dana, who preferred tools to books, then appealed to his father. "Why not let Dana do the plowing? He doesn't like school."

But his father said, "All the more reason for keeping him in school while we can. He'll get his turn at plowing in two years, when he's your age."

Finally Ed yielded. He was up at five o'clock Monday morning to get an early start on the field up the hill near the schoolhouse. All went well until the last bell rang. As he watched the other children file into the schoolroom, the temptation became too strong. He tied the horse to a tree, went in, and took his seat. At noon, after swearing Dana to secrecy, he plowed back down the hill and appeared for dinner. He hurried back to do a few furrows before the afternoon session was called, but only when classes were over for the day did he take up plowing in earnest.

He kept up the deception for several days. Naturally, the work did not progress as fast as his father had expected. When he discovered the reason, he was angry at first, then he relented a little. He could understand, for he didn't like farming either and did it only because of the necessity of providing food for the animals, and to a lesser extent, for the family and for market. Secretly proud of his son's determination, he took over part of the plowing himself and helped to make it possible for the boy to finish the Beaumont school.

Fortunately for the ambitious youngster, a more advanced school, the Monroe Academy, had just been started in Beaumont by a young Presbyterian preacher, the Reverend Charles Canfield. The tuition seems to have been only a dollar a month, and in some way the boy obtained the money and enrolled. In Mr. Canfield he found a friend who was qualified to advise him about his studies and who encouraged him to take such advanced courses as Greek and philosophy.

However, his teacher's interest in the young student seems to have been misinterpreted in some quarters. One evening when the usual group of men sat around the potbellied stove in the store, some wag burst in with, "Say, that Mr. Canfield is trying to do something that God Almighty Himself never thought of doing. He's trying to make a preacher out of Ed Frear!"

It was never clear to me why that was such an unheard-of idea —making a preacher out of a young man as good as (I'm sure) my father was. . . . I do remember his cousin Calla saying, some sixty years later, "Ed was a holy terror in those days." But she refused to explain her disparaging remark, and I never heard such a comment from anyone else. Possibly her attitude was due to the difference in their ages. To a prim little girl, any boy eight years older would probably have seemed a holy terror.

Hoping to find evidence that Calla's charges were unfounded, I turned to the pages of a diary Father kept in the early 1870s. There were good notes on his schoolwork and other employment, and on the weather; his expenses were meticulously itemized— Sunday School collection, 2¢; Lizzie for sweeping floor, 1¢; loaned Henry 3¢. But the account of an evening of fun was, too often to be of any help to me, recorded in Greek.

An entry on his twentieth birthday might be misinterpreted as evidence of guilt, but, knowing Father's tendency toward introspection and soul-searching, I see it as an expression of spiritual hunger. He had recently joined the Presbyterian church. Now he speaks of his weakness and lack of faith, then says: "Twenty years of my life spent, the result of which is registered in eternity.

Until within a few weeks, my time has been spent in sin. Since the first start was made for the better I have often walked far from the right, made many crooked paths. But I am resolved that if, through the providence of God, I am allowed to live twenty years longer, I shall show a better record than the last twenty. . . . Let difficulties present themselves as they may, I will try with God's help to overcome them . . . walk with more reverence toward God and man . . . leaving the past in the hands of a just and true God, and in Him will I trust in time of need. . . . Let the world think as it may. I am not accountable to it."

He seemed to feel that some of his friends thought him queer, or maybe only conceited, but he refused to be influenced by their opinions, for his conviction that he could make something of himself was too strong.

However, his dedication was not to the ministry, for he had early decided to become a doctor. Mr. Canfield encouraged him in this, and with him pored over catalogues to select a school. He also advised him about ways to earn and to save money for school. Here the young man could really use advice, for he was, then and always, a poor manager where money was concerned.

As a student he was interested and conscientious. Years later we found six of his monthly grade reports from the Monroe Academy tucked away among the pages of his diary. Including his grades for attendance, conduct, and diligence—always 100 percent—he made an overall average of 99 percent.

In November following his twentieth birthday, he began to teach. The grades on his teacher's certificate, found with the above reports, were good, with the exception of a "3" in mental arithmetic; we learned from the fine print at the bottom of the page that "3" meant "Middling."

He taught first in Leonard Schoolhouse No. 7 at Lehman, Luzerne County. His salary was thirty dollars a month plus board and keep. "Boarding around" was the standard housing arrangement for teachers in the seventies, and what the system lacked in convenience and cuisine was compensated for by its variety. Father was supposed to spend a week in turn with each of the patrons of the school, but, whether from necessity or choice, he seemed to move about much oftener.

His noon meal was eaten from a dinner pail brought by one of the children. He told us that "lunch was on a by-guess-and-by-golly plan. Some days each and every mother would guess that someone would pack a lunch for the teacher and I'd get none. Then again, by golly, maybe I'd get three in one day."

At the end of his first month of teaching, he took his thirty dollars in pay to Wilkes-Barre and spent more than half of it for schoolbooks for the children, who needed them badly, although they were not his responsibility. He spent three dollars for a clock and bought a school bell.

There was great excitement among the children on Monday morning, and the books were quickly disposed of. A week later he wrote in his journal, "I trusted out all my books and nobody paid me. Yesterday I sent bills for all of them, but today all the satisfaction I got was from one girl who said, 'I would like to have some more books if I could get them. Papa said the bill is all right.'" Later one child, only one, paid for his book.

The following year he taught at Shavertown. The salary was higher, forty-three dollars a month, but it did not include board. He lived at the Shotwell home where the charge, which covered both room and board, was fifteen cents for each meal he actually ate.

Now according to his diary he smoked many "cegars." Then he crossed out the "c" and smoked "segars." One month they totalled a dollar and eighty cents, too much for a boy who was saving for college. Came a day when he spent his last nickel for a segar, then realized what a foolish thing he had done. He smoked that one till it burned his fingers—but he never smoked again.

Writing about his work, he seemed confused about the spelling of "taught" or "tought." He settled for "Teaching." Then appeared the item, "Dictionary, $3.00," so that problem was solved. And he was a good teacher. One entry says, "Co. Supt. Campbell visited school an hour and a quarter. I done well. He gave me praise."

In this school were five big girls. One night he took one of them, Mary by name, home from church—quite a proper thing to do, of course. But next morning Mary came in for a lot of teasing. All the girls whispered and giggled behind their slates and made so much of the incident that the young teacher deemed it best to ignore all the girls outside school hours, and he did. But he had not counted on the fury of a woman scorned, which, when multiplied by five, is considerable. The girls ganged up on him, determined to break up the discipline of the school. And, as he confided to his diary, it looked as if they might do just that.

Things finally quieted down, but it took a lot of praying, both at home and at school, before he had things under control. Now he took no nonsense from his "scholars." In one day he "pulled Olin Shaver from his seat by his hair and gave Chris Gont a lecture." The next day "two boys were punished for shuffling, one whipped for sass."

Without a doubt, the most important day during that winter was January 1, 1876, when he wrote in his diary, "Today I purchased a book on anatomy, and commenced the study of medicine." Mr. Canfield had ordered it for him, and he paid $5.60. This was Saturday—he had walked home from school the night before. He attended Mr. Canfield's wedding, then read anatomy until midnight.

What a temptation that new textbook must have been the next day! But Father never would study on Sunday, nor even read a medical journal. So he attended both the morning and evening services, then walked six miles to Dallas, spent the night with a friend, and next morning walked the remaining mile to his school.

Now he found that if he carefully budgeted his time, he would have six hours daily to read medicine. All went well the first day, although it was eleven o'clock when he closed his book and went to bed. The following night his reading was interrupted at nine o'clock when the stair door opened and Mrs. Shotwell's shrill voice called, "Mr. Frear, it's bedtime. All lights out!"

"But, Mrs. Shotwell, I have started reading medicine," he called down to her, "and my best time is at night. I have so little time during the day."

"Young man," she snapped, "remember this is my house. Bedtime here is nine o'clock."

Reluctantly he blew out the light. The next day he bought a gallon of oil for the lamp and gave it to her, but she was not to be moved. There was to be no sitting up nights. By the end of the week "open war was declared," he wrote. "I am going to study nights, and no one is going to stop me."

After two weeks of arguments that got him nowhere, he moved to the Honeywell home with his cousin, Henry Frear. Here he paid more for board—twenty cents for each meal—but he was permitted to study in peace.

In that day, besides the reading necessary for the young man who aspired to become a doctor, it was usual for him to find a practicing physician who would advise him and direct his studies and also give him some practical experience. This doctor was known as his preceptor. Father found both friend and preceptor in Dr. C. A. Spencer of Dallas, who gave him the use of his library, and also of a skeleton he owned, which was a great help in studying anatomy.

From time to time Dr. Spencer quizzed his protégé on his reading, and whenever possible took him with him on calls. Sometimes this was a definite help to the older man, as when Father "went with Dr. Spencer to set a broken leg for Abram Schultz and later helped the doctor set up a stove."

School closed in March; then he did rough carpenter work, receiving $2.15 for a day of ten hours and paid $.75 daily for board; he often worked overtime, so made a little extra. It was hard work, but it brought closer the time when he could enter medical school.

Then he took a contract which promised greater returns. He was to clear a woodlot, his pay to be the wood it yielded. Working alone so as to make greater profit, he felled the trees and corded the wood. He had a customer ready to buy it; but the night before it was to have been delivered, the wood in some way caught fire and all was destroyed.

Discouraged but not beaten, the young man faced his loss. Payment for the wood would have paid his fare to Iowa; he had chosen the University of Iowa for his medical course. Now he would have to wait a little longer.

He was twenty-five when at last he was ready to leave for Iowa. With him was a friend, George Montross, who also had been born and reared in the Beaumont neighborhood. Arrived in the West, they looked over the country around Sioux City and across the river in Dakota Territory, then came down to Sloan where both found employment, first as carpenters, then as teachers.

By October of the following year, 1880, he had accumulated the few hundred dollars he needed for tuition and for other expenses until he could become established, so he enrolled in the Medical School of the University of Iowa. It was a small school at the time. Only fourteen men were listed on the faculty of the medical department, with about one hundred and fifty students, eight of whom were women. The catalogue boasted: "Students of both sexes are admitted on equal terms and afforded in all respects the same facilities for acquiring a thorough medical education." One woman was graduated in Father's class of forty-five members.

When he entered the school, he had been reading medicine and working with practicing physicians for four years—first with Dr. Spencer, then with Dr. O. N. Ainsworth in Sloan. The advantage of such training was recognized by medical colleges of the day, which made it possible for him to register for the shorter course—a lecture course requiring two years of twenty weeks each. This saved him a year's time and considerable expense, compared to the three-year course, which included class recitations and laboratory work, and which required examinations in all studies at the end of the second and third years.

When one considers the heavy expenses of the medical student of today, it is interesting to note that tuition for this two-year course included a matriculation fee of five dollars, twenty dollars a year for lectures, and a demonstrator's ticket at ten dollars, or a total of thirty-five dollars per year; there was also a final examination fee of twenty-five dollars on graduation. "Hospital Ticket, gratuitous. No charge for material."

Although tuition and other expenses were low, this young student had to practice the strictest economy. A few odd jobs were available, but for one so dedicated to a medical career, his studies demanded every minute of his time; social activities also were definitely limited.

However, there was one notable evening when a fellow student, Dr. Emery Whetstine, invited him to his home. It seems he wanted young Frear to meet the young lady who helped Mrs. Whetstine with the housework and the care of their children in return for her room and board.

This Sue Clemens was a bright, attractive girl, with curly, chestnut-brown hair and deep-set, grey-blue eyes. Sue was ambitious. She wanted to teach, or maybe write, but for either she would need a good education. She was eighth in a family of ten children and her father, though fairly well educated himself, was unable to send her to college, so she was working her own way. All this Dr. Whetstine explained to young Frear.

But Dr. Whetstine had failed to take into consideration Sue's aversion to "medics." They smoked, they drank, they were tough,

23

she said, and no decent girl would have anything to do with them. She was very cool to the young guest, and after acknowledging the introduction, ignored him. When he left she was sitting on the floor amusing the children and did not even look up to bid him good night.

No sooner had the door closed than Dr. Whetstine took Sue to task for her rudeness. "But you know what I think of medics," she said.

"But Dr. Frear is not like the general run of medics," he told her, adding, "He is one of the finest men I have ever known. And I brought him home with me just to meet you."

Sue apologized and promised to be nice to him if he ever came again. She kept her word, and on the next visit the young folks seemed to make up for the bad start their friendship had had. However, it was to be their last meeting for some time, for Sue had to quit school and take her ailing mother to California.

The young student plunged the harder into his studies, for the end of his medical schooling was drawing near.

He seems to have met the required tests for graduation—"Unexceptionable moral character" and satisfactory examination. There was the personal problem of a shabby wardrobe, but Dr. Whetstine kindly loaned him a coat for the graduation exercises. So on March 1, 1882, Dr. Edwin D. Frear, the man who was to become my father, received his diploma. He was now a doctor, his dream a reality.

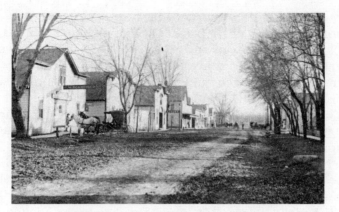

Sloan's Main Street looked, on this early
spring day in the 90's, much like countless
other midwestern small-town main streets.

Chapter 4

THE FIRST HUNDRED DAYS WERE THE HARDEST

W ITH his new diploma, a few textbooks, and such
instruments as he felt were essential, Father went
directly to Salix, a small town about seven miles
north of Sloan, to begin the practice of medicine. Until he could
establish a home and an office, he made his headquarters at the
Duchaine boarding house.

Getting started was slow and discouraging. The town had
a population of a few hundred, and there were said to be fifty
small but prosperous farms within a radius of five miles; he was
the only doctor within this area; still there was little call for his
services.

Most frustrating of all was the lack of maternity cases. He
looked about him at the large families among the Irish and the
Canadian French people who made up the greater part of the pre-
dominantly Catholic community and wondered. Surely not all of
those women depended on midwives from choice. It seemed
there were "babies, babies, everywhere, nor any case for Frear."

But at last a young woman came in and arranged for him to

deliver her baby, due, she said, in two weeks. She was already the mother of two small boys. Determined to be prepared, he sat in his room and read and reread his textbooks on obstetrics; each day he took his shiny, new instruments from his brown leather satchel, checked and polished them carefully, and rewrapped them in their chamois skin cases.

Two weeks passed by without a call from the expectant lady. Three weeks, then a month went by. Then one morning her small son came on a run, stopped only long enough to say, "Ma wants you to come over to our house right away," and he was gone.

Losing no time, Father picked up the leather satchel. A glance inside assured him that all was in order, just as he had left it the night before. He hurried to her house on the edge of town. Answering his knock, his "patient" came to the door with a crying infant, two or three weeks old, in her arms.

"Oh, Doctor," she sobbed. "There's something terrible wrong with my baby! She's been crying like this for hours!"

The young doctor knew a moment of panic. His leather satchel had not the tiniest pill for an infant, and in his haste he had forgotten his medicine case. The baby's cries were frightening for one who, like him, had had little experience with them. Then he remembered hearing Aunt Almi say, "Ain't nothin' wrong with 'em when they can holler like that." So he said calmly, "Suppose you lay her here on the table and undress her, so I can examine her."

The mother slipped off the long nightgown, unfolded the pinning blanket that kept the little feet warm but prevented any movement, removed the three-cornered diaper and the band around her middle, and loosened the shirt. Released from all the trappings, the infant kicked vigorously, then stiffened out and yelled, while Father ran his hand gently over the distended abdomen. He turned her over on her face, and as her weight bore down on her stomach, there was an explosive burp, so sudden that even the baby was startled into a moment of silence; then she resumed her crying, though less noisily.

"What have you been feeding this child?" Father asked.

"Why, I nurse her, Dr. Frear."

"I seem to smell peppermint. Could it possibly be——?"

He called to him a three-year-old who peeked from behind a door, munching candy from a sack. Questioning confirmed his suspicion. The boy had given the baby peppermint candy—"des a teeny piece cause baby got no teef," the boy said.

"I think that explains your trouble," Father said.

"But, Doctor, he couldn't have given her much, and peppermint is a medicine, too."

"Possibly, when it is needed, and sugar is a food too," he said. "But your baby didn't need either one, and the combination was too much for her. I'll send you some pills that will relieve any irritation she may have suffered and I'm sure she will be all right. Let me know if you have any more trouble."

The mother could understand the ailment when reduced to common colic; she was already quieting the baby over her shoulder as the doctor picked up the bag he didn't need, and left.

Gradually work picked up as people got to know him. With fall harvesting there were a few accidents, such as a hand torn in a thrashing machine; there were colds and pneumonia in the winter, some measles in the spring, and cholera infantum as babies wrestled with their second summers. A year after he had come to Salix, he was making a bare living, with collections lagging behind his practice. It wasn't enough; he wanted a home.

He had kept up a correspondence with Sue Clemens and had persuaded her to share his career instead of seeking one of her own. She had returned from California to her home town of What Cheer, Iowa, but that was over two hundred miles away, and he had no money to send for her. After a year and a half of practice it still looked discouraging. And then it happened!

A man hurrying to cross the tracks fell in front of a train and his leg was badly crushed. He was brought to the young doctor, who found it necessary to amputate. His fee for surgery and postoperative care was sixty dollars—and he was paid in cash!

He lost no time, but wired Sue to meet him in Irwin, Iowa, where Dr. Whetstine was practicing, and they were married at the home of their old friends on September 20, 1883.

Father's Salix friends had known nothing of his romance. They had decided that he was girl shy, so were taken by surprise when the young couple arrived by train.

They started housekeeping in a few days in simply furnished rooms. Unfortunately, cooking had never interested Sue, who had planned a career along educational lines; having had four older sisters to help with the housework, she had had little practice at home. So, she told us later, preparing her first meal as Mrs.

Frear was something of an ordeal. Her husband, coming home to dinner, found her in tears, humiliated at having to ask him to eat the badly prepared food.

With understanding so characteristic of him, he took in the situation at a glance. "Say, that looks good," he said. "Come on, let's eat!" Hesitating a little, she poured the coffee and sat down with him.

After a few bites he said, "This tastes mighty good to an old boarding-house bachelor."

When she tried to apologize, he said, "But this is your very first meal. You're doing fine. You'll learn with practice, of course. We've both got a lot to learn if we're to make a success of our marriage, but I'm sure going to enjoy having a home." Thus she was given the assurance she needed to help her to adjust to her new role.

They remained in Salix about three and a half years. My sister Edna was born there on October 4, 1884. Meanwhile, through a series of business deals, Father found himself owner of a store where both drugs and hardware were sold. Not long afterward, he disposed of the hardware stock, possibly influenced to some extent by his experience with a tin peddler.

This man drove up to the store one Friday morning in a spring wagon loaded with tinware. He put on quite an act. He was tired, he said, for he had been on the road all week, and now he wanted to go home. "I drove up from Sloan this morning," he said, "and I haven't covered the country around here. I said to myself, there's a man in Salix who knows a bargain when he sees one, and I came straight to you. Dr. Frear, I'll practically give you that load of tinware if you'll take it off my hands, so I can go home to Sioux City and see my wife and my little baby girl. I got the sweetest little girl, and have to be away from home so much she hardly knows her papa."

The two men exchanged notes about their babies. The astute peddler pretended to be much impressed by Edna's picture and by the stories Father told about her. Then he named a price for the goods. They dickered for a while, and a deal was made. Although they had decided on a lump sum, the peddler made out an itemized list of the articles and prices, and kept a copy with Father's signature affixed.

Father had planned to sell the new stock at a very small profit as a special feature. Customers who came in were plainly interested in the goods and in the prices marked, but invariably they turned away without buying. Eventually, Father learned the reason. After unloading his tinware at the store, the peddler had refilled his wagon and thoroughly canvassed the neighborhood. He had told people that he was selling at wholesale price and showed Father's signed bill to prove it. He had flooded the area with bargain tinware, so that Father's stock was a total loss. He never forgot the transaction, nor the crafty peddler.

After the founding of the Sioux City College of Medicine in 1891, Father became professor of dermatology and hygiene and went to the city weekly; about fifteen years later he established an office there and commuted daily by train—about twenty-one miles. He was constantly being asked to do errands in the city for townspeople. Always glad to help a neighbor, he cheerfully matched dress goods and picked up anything from parts for farm machinery to flowers for a funeral. However, he flatly refused to enter or to have any dealings with a certain store, the now well-established business of the former tin peddler; nor was any member of our family ever permitted to shop there. And Father had considerable satisfaction in knowing that he had deprived the merchant of trade worth many times the cost of a load of tinware.

As for Father's other business ventures, he found that even a drugstore alone presented problems. One day he was returning from the country when he saw an Indian lying beside the road while his pony grazed close by. The man was dead drunk. Father stood for a minute pitying the poor fellow, then he discovered an empty bottle lying beside him. The label was that of a patent medicine known to contain a high percentage of alcohol.

There was only one place he could have bought it—at Frear's Drugstore in Salix, where a clerk was in charge while the doctor was out. It was illegal to sell alcohol in any form to an Indian, and as proprietor, Father could be in for trouble. The Indian stirred and tried to sit up, then settled down for another nap. With the bottle in his pocket, the doctor hurried to town to confront the clerk with the evidence, which, fortunately, no one else had seen. After being properly reprimanded and informed on the law, the clerk was sent to look after the Indian. He carried a bottle of hot coffee, and following instructions, he stayed until the young brave was mounted on his horse and headed for the reservation. There was no further trouble of that sort.

However, Father's greatest trouble was that he was too lenient with customers who wanted credit. He was always reluctant to send out statements. After three years he was glad to sell the drugstore and devote full time to the practice of medicine.

During this time, he was called to Sloan several times by Dr. O. N. Ainsworth, who was practicing there, for consultation or to assist in an operation. So in 1886 he moved to Sloan and the two doctors entered into partnership. His old friend George Montross already had established himself there as a druggist, so that need was met.

Dr. Ainsworth left Sloan to practice in South Dakota about six years later, and Father was left with a fairly large practice. He shared the field with Dr. M. B. Hilts, a graduate of Rush Medical College, who had also come to Sloan in 1886. However, with the long drives in the country required in that day, there was enough work to keep both of them busy. So it was that my father became established in the practice that made up the greater part of his professional life.

I arrived the spring after the move to Sloan. Soon after that the family moved to the six-room, story-and-a-half, L-shaped house, where brother Charley was born in January, 1889, and where we spent most of our childhood. There we had a good home life. We were as comfortable as we could hope to be, living in the nineties in the extremes of the Iowa climate, and we were contented and happy.

Sloan had a good school, and for the most part the townspeople had, like our parents, high ideals for their children. By precept and example we three were led to participate in the religious life of church and community.

Each morning after breakfast, Father read from the Bible and led us in prayer. Mother was more shy and reserved about spiritual things, and when Father was away the little service was omitted. But always after breakfast there was a subconscious reach heavenward, because it was time for morning prayer.

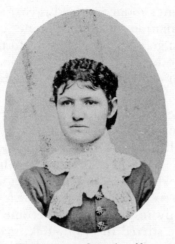

Her dedication as a doctor's wife was Sue Frear's ruling passion. But she also had an ear for music and a love of learning.

Chapter 5

A DOCTOR'S WIFE IN THE NINETIES

A CALL had come for the doctor about four thirty. Slipping a robe over her nightgown, Mother had started a fire while the doctor dressed, and by the time he had hitched up, she had a hearty breakfast ready for him, for this was to be a long, hard trip.

Now it was too late to go back to sleep, so Mother had a long day ahead of her. She could catch up on the housework she had neglected while doing her fall housecleaning, particularly the ironing. She sprinkled down her clothes, then turned to her baking.

The evening before she had made up sponge from her starter yeast. Now she made it up stiff, pounded and kneaded it, and set it aside to rise, then scrubbed the rough, unpainted kitchen floor.

Her next task was a disagreeable one, made so by an annoying habit of the doctor's. Often when making a call he would go

31

directly to the patient's room and lay his coat across the bed while making the examination. Coming home later with but one thought in mind—to get some sleep—he again threw his coat across the bed, theirs. Mother had learned from experience what that could mean for her—and probably for others where he and his coat went.

In vain she pleaded with him, and scolded. "The bed isn't the only place to put a coat. There's always a kitchen chair somewhere. Think of all the work it makes for me."

"All right, all right. I'll remember," he'd promise, really meaning to, but he'd forget. Just the thought of bedbugs made her flesh creep, but as a country doctor's wife she had to face the problem, and a daily inspection had become routine.

That done, she stirred the straw tick, made up the bed, and covered it with a spread made by a patient in payment of her bill. Her pillow shams showed cherubs outlined in red, floating on red-edged clouds. They gave a sense of security to the room with the legends:

Angels sing thee to thy rest.
Angels wake thee—thou art blest.

Now to tidy herself for the day. She twisted her brown hair in a knot high on her head. The short ends that for some women became unsightly scolding locks, curled about her face and neck.

Her gray calico wrapper, the only type of ready-made dress available in Sloan at the time, was floor length, with long, straight sleeves and a high neck; fitted at the waist, it enhanced the figure nature had given her. Many a young woman of the nineties tied her corset laces to the bedpost, then walked away in order to pull herself in to the nineteen-inch waist and hourglass lines so popular at the time. The doctor could, and did at every opportunity, recite a list of horrible things such lacing would do to a woman's health. So it was good that his wife, conceding an inch or two at the waist, found such procedure unnecessary. Too, her cheeks had a rosy glow without being pinched.

Now she dabbed at the shine on her nose with a cornstarch puff, pinned a bit of lace at her throat, took a last look in the mirror, then went to call the children.

We three, Edna, Charley, and I, slept in the room above the kitchen, at the top of the closed-in stairway. We were talking and laughing, and we jumped out of bed when she called. We were always wide awake in the morning, for our health-minded father insisted on a seven thirty bedtime for all three.

We finished dressing by the kitchen stove while she put breakfast on the table. She made up her loaves; at the same time she checked to see that we ate our oatmeal and drank plenty of milk. Soon all were fed, buttoned, and combed. From the sitting room window she watched all three of us in homemade jackets as we left for school; the girls' stubby braids showed below brown velvet hoods; little Charley had his collar turned up, his cap pulled down over his ears, and his hands in his pockets as he braced himself against the wind. We started on a run, but Charley turned and waved at her.

She saw that it had clouded over and a light drizzle was falling—not a pleasant day for the doctor's long trip. By contrast, the sitting room was cheerful and comfortable. She had washed the rag carpet by hand in wooden tubs, one strip at a time, then had sewed them together again while the children carried in straw to cover the floor. They had stretched the carpet while she tacked the edges; then they had skipped and rolled on the puffed-up carpeting while the straw snapped and crackled under their feet. The straw would add warmth to the floor and wear to the carpet.

The wood heater with its isinglass windows had been set up for the winter. Outside, a bank of earth and straw held in place by boards had been thrown up around the base of the house, the better to keep out the cold winds. The house had been made as warm as possible, and as comfortable.

Against the wall stood the red plush sofa; across the room, the spring rocker, with its crazy-patch velvet antimacassar. The melodeon had a bouquet of red paper roses on the round shelf at the right of the keyboard; an oil lamp with a bit of red flannel in the oil for color stood on the left.

The muslin curtains hung crisp and straight. She hoped to get lace curtains and maybe ingrain carpet next year if collections were good—cash collections, that is; to be sure there would be plenty of produce brought in. The farmers shared with the doctor the best their farms had to offer when money was scarce.

There might be a quarter of beef or half a hog at butchering time; after cornhusking there would be plenty of cobs, maybe even corn on the cob, to burn. But you couldn't trade them, or runty pigs, or old hens, or hubbard squash, for luxuries for the home.

She straightened the chenille cover on the walnut center table and raised the hanging lamp; the glass prisms swinging from the shade tinkled musically and scattered bits of dancing color on the wall.

Remembering the time, she went to call the remaining member of the family, the doctor's younger brother, who had come west with them from Pennsylvania. At that time he had been a good looking youth of eighteen, spoiled by his father and older sister, Carrie, who had raised him since his mother's death when he was five. They had planned the trip for him, hoping that the great west and his older brother would make a man of him. As yet, nearly four years later, there had been no miracle of transformation; still he had presented no really serious problems, although the doctor worried constantly because he didn't settle down.

His name was also Charles, but Mother, after slight acquaintance, had called him "the old Nick himself," and the name Nick had stuck.

There was no answer when she called him. "Goodness knows, he could use some sleep," she said half aloud, "and for all he'll do when he gets up, it's hardly worthwhile." Had she cared to, she could have gotten him up very quickly. At one time her nephew, Ernest Smith, had roomed with Nick, and getting the two of them up had proved a problem. But my resourceful mother had worked out an effective alarm system.

Beside Nick's bed was an open drum to let the heat come up from the sitting room below. In the barn Father had two tame ferrets whose job was to keep the grain bin free of rats. One morning Mother placed one of them, Jerry, on a long forked stick, with which she pushed him up through the drum, then under the edge of the bed covers; Jerry headed for a cozy nest beneath them. In seconds he had the bed all to himself. After that she had only to mention Jerry to get the boys wide awake. She held the trick in reserve, but today she would let Nick sleep.

She closed the stair door and filled the stove with wood she had saved for the baking. While the oven was getting hot, then while the loaves took on their golden brown color, she sat humming softly to herself and mended stockings. They were all black:

34

coarse ribbed ones for Charley; finer ribbed ones for the girls; ribless gauze for herself; wool knit socks for the doctor.

The mending done and the bread baked, she laid the ironing board from the table to the back of the chair. She lifted one of the old-fashioned sadirons with a quilted holder, and started with the hardest part of the ironing, the doctor's shirts. He wore the popular (well, not so popular on ironing day) white shirts with stiff bosoms; also the stiff white wing collars. The fashionable celluloid collars were too high for his short neck, unfortunately, for they would have saved ironing seven or more collars every week.

But the shirts were her real problem. She had the first one half-ironed when there was a loud knock at the door. She set the iron on the stove and went to answer. As soon as she turned the knob, a wet wind blew the door wide open. There stood a stocky, ruddy-faced man, warmly dressed from ear-tabbed cap to felt boots. "Good morning, Mr. Johnson. Come on in!" she said, but he declined.

"No, I guess not. I just wanted to see the doctor. He ain't in the office."

"No, he won't be back until noon. Please come inside."

"No, thanks, my feet's dirty, You tell Doc——"

She tried once more. "Don't worry about the mud. If you'll just step inside—it's so cold."

"Oh, I ain't cold." (Naturally not, in his sheepskin-lined coat. She shivered in her cotton dress while he kept on talking.) "Anyhow, I ain't got but a minute. You tell Doc the old woman ain't so good. That pain in her stummick—" and so on, and on, for fifteen minutes. When he finally left and she could close the door she found the fire was out; the house was cold and so were the irons; the half-ironed shirt was dry and had to be dampened so she could start over. But what concerned her most were her aching head and shoulders. She built up the fire and sat with her feet in the oven, her gray shawl pulled close about her, and wondered. Why must people be so inconsiderate? And it would happen again and again all winter—of that she could be sure—while the catarrh she had suffered from since childhood would grow steadily worse.

Presently she got up to finish the ironing. When Nick came down yawning and dragging his feet, she pushed the irons to one side and pulled the coffeepot and heavy skillet to the front of the stove. She glanced at the clock and said, "I suppose you call this breakfast. I'll fry you some eggs." He looked hungrily at the fresh bread, but she laughed and said, "I'm not cutting my warm bread for anybody. Get some bread and the butter from the pantry and bring me your plate."

She served the eggs, then started to iron a pillowcase. "Doctor heard you come in last night, or rather this morning," she said, pausing to look at him.

Nick laughed as he attacked his breakfast. "Did he blow up?"

"No, he turned over and went to sleep. He'd been tossing and listening for you most of the night. Then he was called out at four thirty. He had less than two hours' sleep. This worry is getting him down, Nick. He needs his sleep."

"I'm sorry, Sue, but why on earth should he worry about me?" He got up for more coffee. "Now last night, for instance, a bunch of us got together for"—he hesitated just a second; "for a taffy pull. Certainly no harm in that."

She laughed. "You must have been pretty full of taffy by two o'clock in the morning."

He grinned. "Yep! That's why I left the party so early." He finished his coffee and sat thoughtfully twisting the ends of his mustache. "Well, I'll try to get in early tonight." He looked at the clock. "Gosh! I'm due at the printing office. *The Star* comes out today." He pulled a cigar from his pocket, struck a match on the stove to light it, and hurried out.

She ironed a petticoat with quick, irritated strokes as she thought of Nick. Evidently all he cared about was having a good time, working just enough to keep in spending money; he worked only part time at the printing office.

Fortunately, there was no saloon in town. There had been one a few years earlier; then some of the women, Mother included, decided they didn't want a saloon in Sloan. There was no big campaign with temperance rallies and bottle smashing. The women simply went by twos, took their sewing or knitting, and sat by the hour in the saloon. A few men sneaked to the back door to get their drinks, but there was no meeting with good fellows around the bar, hence less drinking. The saloon keeper found himself unable to cope with the situation, so closed shop.

Naturally, some liquor was brought in from nearby towns, but drinking as a pastime became less popular, so it was easier for young people to gather in homes, where music and clean fun were the rule. Nick with his ready wit, his good voice, and his guitar was always one of the crowd. In a way, his popularity was a blessing, Mother said to herself as she put the ironing board away and started lunch for the children.

At that time she had never heard of peanut butter, canned soups, or prepared cereals, but she had plenty of good bread and butter and wild plum butter—she had put up ten gallons that summer; she fried some potatoes, set out applesauce and a pitcher of milk, and lunch was ready when her two youngest burst in. Edna followed with a schoolmate, Alice Lee. The two girls had been inseparable since they had discovered each other in the first grade. Alice, a pretty child with hazel eyes and dark curls, lived a short distance out of town; she always came home with Edna for lunch. Mother enjoyed their chatter, and laughed with them, but she watched Charley closely. Only five and not a robust boy, he attended the kindergarten that had just been started.

Before she cleared the table, Mother started vegetables for the doctor's dinner. He came home and fell asleep before she had it on the table. He slept for an hour. While he ate, she finished the ironing, then carried the children's clothes upstairs. When she came down he was mixing and heating something in a pan on the stove. "What are you doing with my new saucepan?" she demanded.

"Now, I'm not hurting a thing," he said. "You go on with your work."

"But you're making such a mess! What *are* you doing?"

"Well, I'm trying to make some calomel salve, but it's too runny."

"And you're using lard? No wonder!" She handed him a jar of mutton tallow that she had rendered out to rub on croupy chests. "Try adding a little of this." After a little experimenting, the mixture had just the right consistency. "Now will you admit a woman knows a thing or two, even about a man's work?" she teased.

"Well, I was about to try tallow, but I wanted to give you a chance to show off." He picked up his jar of calomel salve and left.

Soon he was back, with an embarrassed young woman whom he introduced, then he whispered that he wanted a "specimen." She waited on the patient with a cheerful casualness that put her at ease. Since that time urinalysis has become increasingly impor-

37

tant in the diagnosis of disease but has ceased to be the concern of the physician's wife.

Just as rare today is the type of patient who next accepted Mother's hospitality. No dentist being available, the doctor had pulled her abscessed tooth. She was made comfortable beside Mother's kitchen stove in a tilted rocker, and when her sore mouth would permit it, given hot coffee to drink. Her husband called for her later, and they left for a long, cold ride in a lumber wagon.

For the remainder of the afternoon, the doctor's work kept him in the office. At four o'clock school was out, and there were a skinned knee for Mother to dress, a torn coat to mend so it could be worn the next day, and a spelling lesson that needed a workout. Then both the doctor and Nick came home at six, and they all had supper together. Mother had prepared only six meals that day. Sometimes it was more. The supper dishes done, she sat down in the spring rocker to read, but she soon fell asleep. The doctor's wife had had a full day.

The unexpected guest was a common occurrence in our home. If a patient was in the office at mealtime, Father brought him home. Mother, working by the kitchen window, would see them coming across the vacant lot; she could add bread to the fried potatoes, or dumplings to the stew, cut the pie in smaller pieces, or open a jar of fruit; there were always plenty of vegetables.

But sometimes, maybe on washday when the boiler filled with sudsy clothes took up most of the stove, and she had had a hard morning, she would send a child to the office with definite instructions: "Go see if there is anyone in the office with Papa. If he's alone, tell him to come to dinner."

I remember well one unexpected guest. That was the day Papa sued a man for a doctor bill. The case had not come up when the court adjourned for noon recess, and Papa brought the man home with him for dinner. Unknown to our parents, that morning Edna had heard Papa say: "His sisters say he's got the money, but he's boasted he won't pay a cent, so they've urged me to sue. If the judge orders him to pay, he'll be afraid of going to jail for contempt of court and pay up."

Edna had repeated the conversation to Charley and me, adding her own embellishments, and we three had interpreted it in our own way. To us, the man was a criminal, no less. It was our first meeting with a criminal, and we must watch his every word and act. We sat opposite him at the table and stared at him. We whispered behind our hands—and stared. Mother—always the disciplinarian—nudged us under the table, but we failed to understand; we ignored her signal. We still whispered—and stared! It must have been a relief to the defendant to get away from us and have only the court to face.

It was probably the only time Father ever sued for a bill. As I remember it, he got seventy-five dollars, and my Scotch-Irish mother was just the one to spend it so as to get the best possible value.

It was an asset to be Scottish in those early days in Iowa, but the love and laughter of the Irish provided the answer to many a problem. Mother laughed at her troubles, her worries, her shortcomings; when she could without sacrificing discipline, she laughed at her children's pranks. She usually had just the right answer to turn away a personal or annoying question.

I remember when Nannie Williams, a maiden lady in her thirties whose flashing black eyes made one wonder about her demure manner, stayed at our house for a time to be near the office and take treatments.

Little was said about her ailment—it probably wasn't very interesting anyway—but the neighborhood busybody couldn't stand the suspense. One day as I stood in the doorway watching Mother put up strings for her sweet peas, I saw this woman stride into our yard, head thrust forward, long arms swinging. I was reminded of a rodent by her pointed face with her thin lips drawn back from crooked, brown teeth.

She stomped up to Mother without any preliminary remarks, and, accenting each word, she said, "Mrs. Frear! I want to know what ails Nannie Williams!" There was no parrying such a demand. It called for an answer, and Mother was ready with one.

Imitating the woman's tone and inflection perfectly, Mother looked her straight in the eye and said, "Mrs. Bunce! I do not know what ails Nannie Williams!"

Completely taken aback, the woman stared at Mother, snorted her disbelief, and stalked angrily away. Mother just grinned at me and went on with her work. She had told the truth. Of course, she could have told some things about the case, and, adding some details of her own, Mrs. Bunce would have spread it over the neighborhood. But even if Mother had known a big-sounding name and all the symptoms for Nannie's ailment, neither a gossiping neighbor or her own best friend could have pried the information out of her. She knew that, by indulging in gossip, many a doctor's wife had brought professional criticism on her husband and sometimes caused unnecessary suffering for a patient or his family.

Just as disastrous, then as now, was jealousy. Certainly there was opportunity for a young woman to misinterpret the contacts her doctor-husband had with his women patients, especially since some of them were careless or even deliberate in creating wrong impressions. But Mother laughed off many an incident that might have brought on a crisis between people of less sympathetic understanding.

For a time one of Father's patients was a young and attractive divorcee, Molly Burns. Her only source of income was from a farm that she had tried to run by herself after her husband left her. It was hard work for a frail woman, and her health suffered. Unable to get away in the daytime, she always waited until evening, when she could no longer see to work, then came to the office for consultation and treatment.

In our community in the early days, divorced persons were rare and the gossips were obliged to concentrate on poor Molly. So one morning a thin-lipped sister, leaning backward the better to carry her own impeccably righteous load, called on Mother and said, "Mrs. Frear, there is something that your friends all think it's best for you to know. I've come to tell you that Molly Burns comes to town and meets Dr. Frear in his office every night after dark."

Mother had trouble to keep from laughing. "Oh, I've known that all along," she said. "It's all right with me."

Her caller looked horrified and started to speak, but Mother went on: "Last night Molly paid her bill, and I've got the money." She pulled a handful of bills and silver from her apron pocket. "And I'm going downtown and spend it this very day."

The woman left hurriedly, plainly disappointed that her call had ended on such a happy note.

Besides having a sense of humor, Mother enjoyed poetry and music and sang as she went about her work, sometimes softly, sometimes with abandon, depending on her mood.

There was one day in early summer when for the first time we could open all the doors. Outside, birds sang and contented hens visited in the dooryard. Father was setting out tomato plants and a light breeze carried in the fragrance of freshly turned soil. Sunlight streamed across the kitchen floor, and Mother burst into the old song, "There Is Sunshine in My Soul Today!"

Presently a lady from our church came to the door. Without waiting for Mother's greeting, she said, "Mrs. Frear, I'm here to tell you it's your Christian duty to sing in our choir. I've been listening to you all the way from town, and I'm telling you, it was beautiful! We haven't another voice in the church half as good."

Mother's response to that announcement was a hearty laugh. Then she said, "I'm so glad you told me. I'll try not to make so much noise after this so as not to disturb the town. But you know very well that I seldom can get to church, let alone go to choir practice."

Mother attended church whenever possible, but she could never count on going. Many farmers who would not think of working in the fields on Sunday failed to consider the doctor's need of rest; since the team was not being used in the fields, they would drive in to see the doctor and have him look at Johnny's wart, or dress a bad burn that hadn't healed, or give the wife something for that awful cough.

Mother felt she must be home to take messages or talk with patients who came. And if the doctor had had a hard night she might try to devise some way to avoid or postpone a consultation so the doctor could sleep. And on Sunday as well as on a weekday, a compress or an arm sling might be needed; the obstetrical instruments might have to be cleaned and boiled after a delivery; the doctor might need hot water, and sometimes this alone posed a problem. Wood was scarce in that part of Iowa, and the soft coal brought in was limited in supply and high priced.

Possibly my memory is distorted by the feel of the old bushel basket that bumped against my knees as I carried it, overflowing, from corncrib to kitchen; but we seemed to burn corncobs most of the time. I remember too that we sometimes twisted hay into ropes, then tied them in knots for fuel. There were special stoves —hay burners—for utilizing the prairie grasses, and one still heard of burning buffalo chips, but my childhood was spent, one might say, in the corncob era.

Regardless of the fuel problem or the heat of summer, Mother

41

was seldom caught without hot water when it was needed. However, it was working beside her husband in an emergency that gave her the most satisfaction. She knew instinctively how to ease a patient's position, massage a back, or stimulate circulation in a bed-weary limb. Many a newborn baby was placed in her arms, and the first sound to meet his pink ears would be Mother's voice whispering sweet nothings as she dressed him to meet his world.

At times situations called for a special kind of courage, when so little could be done and she must forget the tremendous need that could not be met. One early summer morning Father returned from a call on a young woman who lay dying of abdominal cancer in a two-room cabin near the railroad track. As usual, he called as he came in, "Sue? Oh, Sue! Where are you?"

She came in from the entry where she was straining the morning milk. Seeing that he was distressed, she asked, "What's wrong? Is she gone?"

"No. Not yet, poor soul," he said. "But it can't be long now, twenty-four hours at the most."

"Who is with her?" she asked, sensing a need.

"Only her husband. Her sister is coming this afternoon. The two children are with neighbors. They came in to help at first, but one after another they've given up. You can't really blame them." He poured a cup of coffee, but set it down and walked back and forth across the floor. "Oh, it's awful, Sue. The stench—flies swarming all over her—and she cries and moans when she is conscious—which isn't often now, thank God. I've given her all the morphine I dare. I don't know what more I can do."

Mother washed the strainer cloth while he talked. "Her husband isn't much help. Just sits with his head in his hands. I roused him up to keep the flies away from her when I left." He sat down to drink his coffee.

Mother opened the trap door in the kitchen floor and carried the crock of milk down the steps to cool on the cellar bottom. Returning, she scribbled on a piece of paper. "I'll leave a note for Edna. She and Alice can put the lunch on," she said.

Father spoke quickly. "I can't ask you to go over there, Sue."

She said, "You haven't. But she needs someone with her." She tied on a clean apron and reached for her sunbonnet. "Come on. I'm ready."

She found conditions even worse than she had expected. She had all she could do to keep patient and bed clean, shoo flies (with strips of paper tied to the end of a stick), wipe the poor drooling mouth, and pray—for what, she hardly knew. In late afternoon relatives came by train, and she went home, depressed by a sense that she had failed.

They came for Father before daybreak next morning. When he returned later, quiet and tense, she knew without asking that the end had come. She knew too what was in his mind. She said, "You did everything possible for her, all anyone could do."

"I know, but it wasn't enough," he said sadly. "Someday they'll find a cure for cancer. I hope it won't be long." He looked out the window, then said, "I think I'll go out and hoe the potatoes while you get breakfast on." Her eyes followed him; she smiled at the energy he put into his work. There his tension would disappear and his spirit be renewed for another day's work.

She heard the bell on the Methodist church toll to announce the death, its muffled tones marking the age of the deceased. Mother counted them as she fried golden slices of cornmeal mush. Only thirty years old! Long folds of black crepe would fall from the doorknob of the deceased's home. Her husband might wear a band of crepe on his sleeve—it wasn't always done although a widow would certainly wear a black dress and long crepe weeds. (Father deplored them as a hindrance to a woman's health and to her mental and spiritual adjustment.)

The funeral would be in the church, of course. There would be few flowers, possibly some from neighbors' gardens. Mother decided to pick all her sweet alyssum and make a wreath for the altar. Right now she must call the doctor to breakfast and start another day, with its many possibilities.

Mother's interest in his patients was a source of great pride for Father; for her, the sympathy and understanding toward his work gained from her relations with them added much to the richness of her life.

Sometimes mothers would leave their children with her while they consulted the doctor, then did a little shopping. A baby might be left to lie on her clean bedspread (with plastic panties unknown) for an hour—or half a day. She welcomed them all for she loved children, especially babies.

But occasionally the older children overplayed their welcome. One young mother of three, who lived in town while a patient of Father's, had found the brief interlude without her children so enjoyable that she started dropping them off at our house whenever they became a nuisance, and this happened increasingly often.

One day the five-year-old boy set a kitten on the hot stove "to see him dance." Later, Mother, investigating meows and cries, rescued a half-suffocated kitten from the oven. On her return the mother found her son securely strapped in a chair and was informed that, for her offspring, the door would remain definitely and permanently closed. Mother loved animals, and to abuse them was not to be tolerated.

Father, too, loved animals. On one occasion his fondness for cats could have gotten him in serious trouble. It was cold, and a heavy snow had fallen, when he took the sleigh for a five-mile drive north of town. He returned about noon and took an unusually long time to stomp his boots and shake the snow from his fur coat before coming in. He tossed his coat on a chair and asked, "Have you got some hot coffee?" Mother set the coffeepot on the stove.

He stood there warming his hands. Soon there was a meowing and scratching at the back door. Father was there so soon one might suspect he was waiting for the summons. "Well, well! Look here, Sue!" he said. " 'The wicked wandereth abroad for food.' Have you got any food for the wicked?" He set a scrawny, mangy black kitten on the floor.

Mother looked suspiciously from him to the emaciated animal, but she produced a saucer of table scraps. "All right, Wicked, eat, then please go home." She picked up Father's coat and started to spread it out to dry.

Father took it from her. "Never mind that coat. How about the coffee?"

But Mother had noticed something. She pointed to a jagged tear in the back of the coat. "How in the world did you do that?"

"Oh, that? I must have snagged it a little."

"Snagged it a little? Doctor, that tear is over a foot long! I want to know what happened," she demanded.

"Sue, don't nag me. I just got home from a long, cold trip. What I need is a cup of hot coffee." He sounded almost pathetic.

She filled a cup, stirred in sugar and cream, and handed it to him. "There's your coffee. Now! Where did that cat come from?"

He dodged the question. "Don't you ever read Job? 'The wicked wandereth abroad——' "

44

"Humph!" she interrupted. "Job had nothing to do with this. You picked this cat up someplace." She half-suspected the truth, even before she wormed it out of him next day.

About three miles out of town he had heard pitiful cries and thought it might be the voice of a lost child. He stopped to listen, then discovered this kitten, caught in the crotch of a tree, about ten feet above the ground, on the other side of a barbed wire fence. He tried to go on and leave it, but couldn't.

It was too cold to remove his coat and felt boots; it would be hard to get through the fence with them on, then climb the tree far enough to reach the kitten—but that's what he had done. Then, holding the clawing kitten, he had had trouble getting back through the fence, and his coat had caught on the wire.

"You've no right to take such a risk at your age," she scolded.

"Sue, I couldn't have slept a wink with that cat on my conscience," he said earnestly.

"And if you'd fallen from the tree and broken your leg, I suppose you'd have slept just dandy, lying there on the ground until someone found you, a day or so later." Mother's patience was exhausted. "Well, we don't need any more cats. You can just find a home for him."

But no one wanted Wicked. Moreover, he seemed to like it with us, which wasn't too bad, until he started taking the best chairs for his naps, stealing the kittens' food or jumping on the dining table for snacks, and using the far corner of the bedroom closet for his private sandpile.

Father would make excuses for him when reminded that Wicked was his cat, until he started biting and scratching patients who came to the door; now there was no alternative—Wicked had to go.

Father said, "Chloroforming will be the most humane method; I'll take care of it." But he dreaded it and procrastinated. until Mother set three o'clock on a certain day as a deadline.

At the appointed hour, she said, "We are all ready. Wicked is down cellar in a washtub covered with boards weighted down with bricks."

Father went to the office for chloroform. Returning, he handed her a large wad of cotton and a bottle that he said contained enough chloroform to kill three cats; he added sheepishly, "Sue, I'm really sorry I can't stay and do this, but Bert Owen was

45

in the office waiting for me, and I've got to go over there. I'll be back by five, if you'll just wait——"

"I've done all the waiting I'm going to," she snapped. "I'll do it by myself."

She saw the expression of mixed guilt and relief as she turned away, but she was so angry that nothing could stop her now. With the cotton tied around a slender stick, she soaked it well with chloroform and pushed it between the boards in front of the feline nose, only to find the nose was somewhere else. She probed, he jumped. Wicked was neither ready nor willing to meet his Creator, and since the crack was straight and narrow, and the tub was round and wide, he had the advantage as he tore madly about his small prison and yowled, spit, and scratched.

When he raised the boards a few inches, she tried to hold them down with her hands, and the bottle fell and rolled across the floor, spilling most of the contents. She sat on the cover and looked around for something to use as a weight, but nothing was within reach; she sat still trying to figure out a way of escape. No one would hear if she called for help. There were the cellar steps and the door at the top, but, with old Wicked shoving and clawing frantically, if she took her weight off the boards for an instant he would jump out and tear into her. For the present she must stay right where she was.

She was cold, and the musty odor from the bins of stored vegetables was oppressing; but above all she was nauseated and drowsy from the fumes of the chloroform. She must stay awake at all costs; maybe Wicked's yowling would help there.

After an hour she heard the sound of running feet—school was out. She called to us, and there we found her, weeping, pale, and weak from nausea and nervous exhaustion. Charley cried from sympathy, first for her, then for the cat, while Edna and I offered to help finish the task, but she said, "No, thanks! That pleasure belongs entirely to your father." Together we lifted a sack of potatoes onto the cover of the tub and left Wicked there.

Mother went to bed and lay with her face to the wall. No one spoke when Papa opened the door and called, "Sue? Oh, Sue! Where are you?" He looked at our long faces as we stepped from the bedroom. He hurried to her calling, "Sue! Answer me, what's wrong?" She neither moved nor spoke, but she let him feel her pulse.

He appealed to us children, but we only kept quiet until

Edna suggested, "You might look in the cellar."

Wicked started a wild fight, but Father dealt a blow to his head which quieted him until the lethal dose could be administered. The end was total. Poor Wicked did not even live on in the affection of his family.

Mother was humiliated by her failure. Later, when she could talk about it, she said a doctor's wife should know how to chloroform a cat, or have sense enough not to try.

Mother's dedication as a doctor's wife was her ruling passion, and its major expression was in sharing the doctor's hopes and plans for their children. They must have a happy home life, with both affection and discipline, and strong, healthy bodies. They must have the education she had missed and for which he had struggled so hard. She carried a full share of this responsibility.

She taught us girls to do housework and sewing and expected us to do our share, but if there was something to do for church or school, that came first. She did the work gladly while we studied, went to church, rehearsed for a program, or even went to one of the few parties held in our town. She helped us to memorize poems and songs, and if we took part in a program, she always managed to attend.

She shared with us her joy in creating things both lovely and practical. We made countless dresses for our dolls, so slipped easily into sewing for ourselves, even to the lined and fitted skirts of seven gores worn when we were fourteen and sixteen years old. Mother herself revelled in making pieced quilts, as well as feather-stitched crazy-quilts and antimacassars. In her hands, seven tomato cans covered with heavy woollen material—probably a discarded pair of trousers—were joined together to become an attractive hassock, padded on top and brightly embroidered.

I'll never know how Mother found the time for handicrafts and needlework, with all the housework she had to do, besides helping Father when he needed her. And still there were times in the winter when, with the supper work done, the children in bed, and Father out on a call, she had an evening alone to spend as she pleased. At such times she often sat down at the organ and played and sang the old songs she loved.

I remember one night when I lay awake listening to the plaintive strains of "Sunset Reverie." I slipped out of bed and went into Nick's room—he was out for the evening—to lie on the floor beside the open drum so that I could hear better.

47

Presently she played "The Bridge" and began to sing, softly at first; then as she yielded to the sweetness of the hour, my mother's voice floated up to me in full, rich tones. "Juanita" followed, then "Ben Bolt."

But the song that brought tears to my eyes was "I'll Take You Home Again, Kathleen." In childish imagination, I pictured my mother as the bonnie bride. I wondered about the place "where your heart has ever been," and whether Papa would take her back again "across the ocean wild and wide." Could it be that Mamma wasn't happy with us? And was it because we children were so bad?

Lying there with my feet curled up in my nightgown, I thought of how hard Mamma worked to take care of us, and I remembered many times when I had been naughty. I'm sure I wasn't a really bad child, but little acts of disobedience stood out pretty big as I listened to my mother's voice. I buried my face in my arms and cried.

When I heard her close the organ and sit down in the squeaky rocker, I slipped down the cold, dark stairway, and across the bare kitchen floor to the sitting room. She held out her arms to me and wrapped me in her gray shawl. With my arms around her neck, I sobbed, "Mamma, will you forgive me for being such a naughty girl? Please, Mamma, I'll be good. I promise. I want you to be happy so you'll stay with us." She must have been puzzled by that last statement, but I was promptly forgiven, and warmly loved. And I was reassured by her tenderness as she took me upstairs and tucked me in bed.

I promised to go right to sleep if she'd sing one more song— "I Think When I Hear That Sweet Story." As her voice drifted up to me, I thought that my mother's singing must be the most beautiful music in the world. As I grow older, I am inclined to think that I was right.

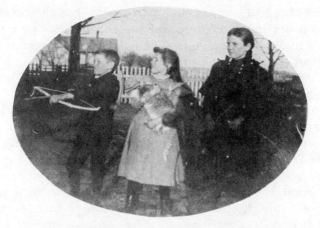

Lively imaginations turned a small-town childhood into an adventure for Charley (7), Cora (9), and Edna (11)—and their parents.

Chapter 6

THE DOCTOR'S CHILDREN

I SUPPOSE Father's office in the year 1900 would in many ways fall short of modern standards, but it had a great fascination for us three children. We would have been uncomfortable in today's spotless, air-conditioned waiting rooms, and awed by equipment so complicated, so obviously sterile. Come to think of it, I don't see children of today playing in their father's office. Could they be missing something?

However, Father's office appealed to each of us in a different way. Edna, as a small child, had a secret longing to be a patient and sit in the big leather chair in the consultation room. Such a wonderful chair! It could be raised or lowered, flattened out or set upright, with the footrest and headrest at various angles. What a thrill to have Papa adjust the chair just right, then take her pulse, and have her say "A-a-a-h," always with a worried look on his face.

And that is where Papa found her one morning when she was

seven, and about to lose her last baby tooth. For the occasion she had put on her best dress and, she hoped, the look of one about to die. Actually, that pallor was achieved by a generous application of Mother's cornstarch puff.

"What in the world are you doing there?" Father asked when he had recovered from his surprise.

"I got an awful bad tooth. Maybe you'll have to give me chloroform."

"Chloroform?" he repeated. "Oh, come now! It can't be that bad." He reached for her but she clung to the arms of the chair.

"You better take my tempashur. I feel awful bad."

He pried her loose from the chair and sat down with his knees spread apart, still holding her hand. "Just let me take a look at it first."

She hung back, but he pulled her close, clamped his knees together to hold her, and picked the tooth out easily with his fingers. "That didn't hurt a bit, now did it? See? You're all right." But the usually stoical Edna burst into tears and ran sobbing from the office, leaving a puzzled father, who couldn't possibly know that the child's heart was broken because her carefully planned drama had been ruined.

To me, that chair was rather frightening. I spent more time in the office than Edna did, and heard too many groans and cries coming from that room. But I liked to be with Papa and to imagine that I was helping him. I'm sure he invented things for me to do, just to keep me near him. Too, I liked to talk to people who came in the office, and as I grew older, I loved to hold babies or amuse children while their mothers consulted with Father.

Charley was always interested in the shiny instruments and in the odd-shaped boxes and bottles. He would ask, "Papa, can I have this when it gets old?" and Papa would inquire, "What do you want it for?" He probably hoped his son would say he wanted to play doctor, but Charley always answered, "I wanna make sumping wiv it."

Charley did play doctor sometimes in our playhouse in the woodshed. I was always the mamma, and kittens dressed in doll clothes were the children. Charley was both papa and doctor. He gave the children flour-and-water medicine, colored with beet juice, mixed in bottles Father had given him. He never lost a patient.

For more active exercise, we had a swing and a trapeze in

the corncrib, and we played hide-and-seek in the barn and hayloft. All buildings were large enough to hold the hay, feed for the stock, or corncobs, which might come in all at once as they were harvested. Hardly classified as medical equipment, such buildings were still a necessity for the country doctor.

The pigpen too was in demand, as when Sig Lund brought in three weaner pigs on account. It never occurred to us children that pigs made nice pets, but we accepted Father's offer to give each of us one to feed and care for, with the promise that we would get the money for them when sold.

Charley, who was eight at the time, had some scheme in mind that required money—possibly at that time it was to buy a Shetland pony. Anyway, his piglet got excellent care, and even learned his name. "Inky" would come squealing to the fence to have his back scratched with a corncob or to get an extra snack of bread and milk.

As he was leaving on a call one day, Father asked the hired man to sell the best of the pigs. This man, Jerry Murphy, had been a tramp a year earlier, and because he had a skin infection, someone had sent him to Father. His gratitude when the eruption was cured and his loyalty to Father were unquestioned; further, he knew Father needed the money. But he had watched Charley work with his pig, and his warm Irish heart was touched by the boy's grief when Inky was taken away. He returned from the market and laid the money in Charley's hand.

Eleven dollars and seventy-three cents looked pretty big to the youngster; it even eased the impact of his grief. He strutted proudly and showed his wealth to all who would look. For the time Father had forgotten the deal he made when he gave us the pigs. Reminded of it, he pretended real enthusiasm for Charley's good fortune. Then he made a proposition.

He explained interest on loans to the boy, and offered to pay him 6 percent for the use of his money, so that in a year he would have almost twelve dollars and a half. "That's the way many rich men got their start," he said. "You can see, can't you, how your money would grow?"

Charley listened carefully, then said, "Yes, Papa, I can see that all right. But wouldn't it be safer in the bank?" And that's where his money went.

It was hard to be firm with Charley since so much of the time he was ill or convalescing. Father must have wondered at times whether his son would ever reach manhood and be able to study medicine. As an infant he had pneumonia. At two he developed a large ringworm on his head after showering affection on a stray kitten. For months he wore a fitted muslin cap tied under his chin to protect the ringworm and to keep from spreading the infection.

At nine he suffered an attack of rheumatic fever, with St. Vitus dance—so severe that for a time he could neither talk, nor swallow when he was fed. Measles and scarlet fever each took a turn. The summer he was fourteen he tried working on a farm about forty miles from home. Father knew and approved of the family; one son was a third year medical student. But when Charley contracted mumps, they made light of it and let him walk four miles to the station to take a train for home. He arrived with a raging fever and had no recollection of how he got there.

But patience and good care from both parents brought the boy through a happy childhood, even with some participation in sports. His enthusiasm for baseball at one time worried Father. When he learned that Charley didn't have what it takes to make a professional baseball player, he seemed to be unable to decide whether to be sorry his son wasn't good enough, or to be glad the temptation was removed.

Charley helped care for the horses and rode them occasionally, but what he really wanted was a dog. Most dogs in town were his friends and often followed him home. One stray refused to leave and Father reluctantly consented to letting him stay. The grateful mongrel went all out to protect us from intruders. The first man to come for Father in the night couldn't get past Bowser to ring the bell. He started around the house to get away, stepped into a hole the dog had made, and fell. Bowser's barking awakened Father; he found the man more angry than hurt, but Charley's first and only dog had to go.

During his illnesses Charley had read and been read to till he had gained a love of good books. At ten he enjoyed such books as *The Leather-Stocking Tales, Ivanhoe,* and *Les Misérables.*

Having no comics or western movies to influence his taste, he had little interest in guns. This was good, for Father had seen many gunshot wounds, and he never for a moment relented in his objection to firearms. Even the danger of a chance coyote coming on the place did not, in his opinion, excuse having a loaded gun in the house. Toy guns were not tolerated, or even sticks used in play for shooting games. Nor did one of us dare to point a finger at another and say, "Bang!" There could hardly be an accidental shooting by one for whom such precaution had become instinctive, as it had in this doctor's children.

So this small boy had no toy pistol in fancy holster hanging from his belt. However, there was no objection when he made his own bow and arrow. And when, after reading *Ivanhoe*, he was interested in fencing, Father let him have foils, possibly to encourage exercise. There was no one to teach him to fence, and he had no opponent; we girls refused to be the victims—those foils were not toys. But no youngster of today gets a more realistic thrill from his "Bang! Bang!" than Charley did when he lunged at an imaginary foe and shrilled out, "Tou-ché!"

Then someone gave him a copy of *Peck's Bad Boy*. Here was a new kind of character, one into whom he could readily project himself. He tried to emulate the bad boy with a swaggering walk, insolent speech, and mischievous pranks. But impudence was never tolerated in our household, and when Mother caught him soaping the front walk, she made him scrub it all off. Then Father learned that Charley had accused the grocer of weighing in his thumb and selling wormy cheese, and he started an investigation. The offending book was discovered and confiscated. Charley searched for it for a few days and found it—under Father's pillow!

Our activities were not greatly restricted so long as we didn't take too great chances. We could climb trees to our hearts' content. One limb on the ash tree by the fence was worn smooth and shiny from our skinning the cat.

Our duties increased at the office as well as at the house as we grew older. We swept and dusted; later we built the fire. On one occasion, at least, that could have brought on trouble.

One morning while Father was at breakfast, a middle-aged couple came to the house. I told them he would be in the office very soon and went with them to unlock the door. Since the morning was cool, I built a fire. It took only a few minutes to start the air-tight heater, then I shut off the drafts and returned to the house. Father went out soon after, but almost immediately he was back, calling excitedly for me. "How close were you to those people?" he asked.

"Oh, half across the room," I said. "I started the fire, then left. Why?"

"Because they're both broken out with smallpox," was his worried answer.

This was during my high school years and I had previously been exposed to smallpox without getting it, so we were not too worried; still we took every precaution, and I did not contract the disease.

One of our earlier tasks was to roll bandages. These were torn from old sheeets and rolled in a box Father had rigged up, with a rod and a handle to turn. If the finished rolls were not as sterile as the ones in use today, at least they were clean by nineteenth century standards, for both the sheets and our hands were washed with good old brown, homemade soap.

We were expected to know most of the patients who came in by name, and sometimes we visited with them, but we must never say, "How are you today?" since that might remind one of his illness and encourage him to discuss his symptoms, and that was bad. Nothing heard or seen in that office was ever to be repeated or discussed outside; we must not even tell who had been in. Many a gossip who tried to get information from us found the "doctor's kids" tight-lipped even to the point of rudeness.

The office took on a new interest sometime in the early nineties when Father bought what was about the latest thing available for the treatment of rheumatism. It must have had a proper name, but we just called it "the battery." It was a hand-operated generator encased in a polished oak box a little larger than a shoe box. One turned a crank to generate a current; the harder it was turned, the stronger the current. Attached by cords were two cylindrical electrodes which could be held in the hands, and it took but a small charge to tighten the muscles so it was impossible to let go.

The electrodes could be replaced with attachments for massaging a neuralgic face or rheumatic back—the purpose for which it was intended—but this did not interest us children. Papa let us hold the electrodes while he turned gently. We giggled at the tingling sensation, squealed as our hands tightened, then yelled for him to stop. He even let us try it on each other, under his watchful eye, and enjoyed it as much as we did. So we shared his pride in the new possession, which he left on the waiting-room table for a few days where it could be seen and demonstrated to anyone interested.

Edna was about seven at the time. Always quick with things

mechanical, she was intrigued with the possibilities of this new device. It happened that she was in the office when Jim Williamson, whom she knew well, came in to see Father, and while he waited she showed him the new battery.

"Want to see how it works?" she asked. "Here, hold these and I'll turn." She started slowly as Father had done. "Does that hurt?"

Jim smiled. "No, it just tingles a little."

"All right," she said, turning faster. "Now does it hurt?"

He forced a laugh. "Not much, but I don't think we'd better play with it any more." He tried to lay the electrodes down.

"Now you can't let go!" Edna laughed, still turning.

He was getting worried. "I'll tell you, Edna, I think we'd better stop now. You might break Papa's nice new battery, and what would he do to you then?"

"Oh, I won't break it. I can run it lots harder. Watch!"

She turned faster. Now he was unable to protest; he could only utter queer sounds and make funny, pop-eyed faces. And when she turned still faster, he fell to the floor, and lay there twisting and writhing convulsively. Edna thought it a good show, and her shouts of laughter disturbed Father so that he came to the door to quiet her. Alarmed by what he saw, he sprang across the floor and jerked the child's hand from the crank.

With a groan, Jim sat up. Father helped him to a chair and massaged his cramped muscles. When Jim could find his voice, he blurted out, "Doc, she might have killed me!"

Only then did Edna realize the seriousness of what she had done. She backed toward the door, arms tight against her sides, fingers spread, eyes bulged with fright. Suddenly Father turned to her. "You git for home fast as ever you can and stay there till I can 'tend to you!" Edna heard the first two words. Without waiting to hear more, she "gat."

Later I heard Father tell Mother about it. He chuckled in spite of himself, as he often did over Edna's pranks. Mother asked, "Could that kill a man?"

"I doubt if that generator is strong enough," he answered. "She turned it about as hard as it would go. I don't know if a man could be much more scared than he was, and live. I'd hate to take that chance myself."

Needless to say, the battery was removed to a place out of reach of children—an unnecessary precaution so far as Edna was concerned. In fact, she avoided the office for some time, and seemed to prefer to play with Charley and me.

She was a lot of fun, too, although she did tease us. Once she told us that if we'd leave a horse hair in the rain barrel, after a while it would turn into a snake. We didn't stop to think that we didn't want a snake—we tried it. After what seemed a long time, we took it out and examined it for snaky features, but found none. "You took it out too soon. Now you'll have to get a new horse hair and start all over," she told us. We tried again and again, waiting longer each time, but the result was the same; winter came, the rain barrel froze over, and we gave it up.

One day she begged me for a piece of pie I had saved from dinner, but I refused. "All right, you'll be sorry," she said; "If you eat it you'll get a black moustache." Sure enough, next morning my upper lip bore a heavy black streak.

Edna had put it on, of course, with black cork. "And I had an awful time with it," she said. "Every time I touched your lip, you wiggled it like a rabbit's nose, and I had to stop and laugh."

However, when necessary, Edna could put her clowning to good use. One afternoon when we came home from school we found that Mother had gone to help Father with an emergency case, and they had not returned. She had left a note for Edna with instructions to follow in case she was late, but had not foreseen that they would be delayed for hours. About five o'clock it grew dark and Edna carefully lighted the oil lamp. We had never been alone after dark before, and we were afraid. Charley was only five, and he cried for Mamma. Edna tried in every way she knew to distract him. She made funny faces and turned somersaults. Then she settled him on the sofa beside her and read to him, but whenever she stopped for breath he demanded more, and cried if left to his own thoughts.

Her next stunt was to stand on her head with her back to the organ, and while she pedaled with one hand, she played a tune on the organ with her heels. Charley laughed until he cried. But she couldn't hold that position long, so she made up stories to tell him, and silly songs, until both Charley and I almost forgot we were afraid.

The folks came home at six thirty. Charley ran into Mother's arms, but Edna threw herself on the sofa and sobbed. We had not realized it, but Edna had been even more frightened than we younger children were; the strain and her responsibility for us had been almost too much for her.

As Edna and her friend Alice approached high school age, they found many things of extracurricular interest, which they often shared with their schoolmates, much to the annoyance of their teachers. Of course, they explored the rich source of material in Father's office.

On a trip to Sioux City, a dentist had asked him to take an upper plate to be delivered to a patient in Sloan. Edna discovered it and found she could slip it over her own upper teeth; so, encouraged by Alice, she wore it to school. Needless to say, she was sent home—to find Father feverishly hunting for the denture.

After a few such incidents, most of them amusing rather than harmful, Father found the girls one day experimenting with a bottle of chloroform, taking turns inhaling the contents to see how long they could stay awake; whereupon Father put a definite and immediate stop to their office explorations.

When he heard the girls were whispering and giggling in church, he faced a different problem. He could seldom get away from the office to go to church, and when he did, usually someone came for him, which embarrassed him and disturbed the service. But this situation called for action. Leaving instructions that he was to be called only in an emergency, he started for church with Edna and Alice the following Sunday.

The reason for his attendance was rather obvious, so when the trio entered the church, some people smiled, and a muffled titter was heard when he made Edna move over so he could sit between them. Then it happened! Just as the prayer ended, an usher tapped him on the shoulder. Mrs. Agnew was in labor, and Father knew that in this case there might be serious complications.

Between rows of smiling faces, the embarrassed doctor walked to the door and left the two girls, and many adults as well, trying to control their laughter. So, attending church with the girls was not the solution. An appeal to their sense of fairness brought better results. After all, they agreed, there were plenty of places outside church to have fun.

Our parents had such high ideals for their three children who showed no special aptitude, character, or charm. It must have been discouraging at times, but they kept trying. Discipline was important; we must learn to work and become useful citizens; our education, hopefully, was to include college, but it must be comprehensive as well, so we must have at least a taste of the arts.

As a part of his plan, one summer Father arranged for us girls to take painting lessons from an elderly patient whose work he had admired. She lived two miles in the country, but he promised to take us out. He would have, of course, but it seemed that at lesson time he was always out on a call. So we would start out on foot and accept the first ride offered. Everyone knew us; no one passed us by. We went by buggy, surrey, cart, lumber wagon, and once we rode on top of a load of hay.

Just as graciously offered was a ride in the butcher's wagon. We rode standing in the back, jostled and bounced about as the heavy wheels fought the clods and ruts of baked gumbo. It would have been easier to walk than it was to keep our balance in the slat-enclosed body (not by Fisher), that on the return trip would carry some pampered steer from farm to slaughterhouse.

After all our time and effort, some spark of genius should have emerged. Not so. Nor was there any urge on our part for self-expression by brush or crayon. At the end of the summer, when each had completed two amateurish paintings, the lessons were discontinued.

Mother had approved of the try at painting, but she was more interested in music. She had already started Edna on the organ when she was eight. And what's more, she kept her on the schedule exacted by teachers in the nineties—one full hour of un-interrupted practice daily. For a bundle of energy and mischief such as Edna, that was a big order.

I learned something of Mother's system one day when I came in and found her ironing, with a tin pan and a few dishes lying on the table close at hand. From behind the closed sitting room door came the strains of Edna's first two-hand piece, and as she played she sang the words:

> Go tell Aunt Rhoda . . . her old gray goose is dead,
> One she'd been saving . . . to make a feather bed.

As she finished the piece, she stopped, obviously listening.

Mother winked at me, picked up the dishes and rattled them; Edna resumed her practice. Mother laid the dishes down, laughing, and said, "She'd rather practice than wipe dishes, and when she thinks they're done she'll want to quit. Now don't you tell on me." I kept her secret, and she kept up the sound of wiping dishes for an hour each day, so that Edna did very well with her music.

By the time she entered high school, Edna was playing for the singing both in school and Sunday school, and playing solos for special occasions. We were obliged to provide our own entertainment in the nineties—not even the nickelodeon had reached Sloan —so church and school programs were popular.

The highlight of the year was Christmas Eve, when each of our three churches had its own festivities. In the Methodist church, Edna took part in the music and I usually "spoke a piece." Charley was too shy to appear before the public. A large fir tree was imported for the occasion. We trimmed it with paper cutouts and chains, strings of popcorn and cranberries, and real, lighted candles. A kind Providence must have watched over us, for we never had a fire. Then too, gifts for the children were brought and put on the tree.

However, no gifts for us three children from our parents ever found their way to the tree, because of Father's strong objection to the practice. Montross's drugstore was the center of Christmas shopping; there Father saw parents come in and spend money that he, as their family physician, knew was needed for medicine, as well as for nourishing food, clothing, and household comforts. (Did he think, too, of doctor bills?)

Many would buy toys, games, and trumpery until they reached the limit of both cash and credit, then load the spoils into the lumber wagon and carry them home. Early Christmas Eve they were again piled into the wagon and taken to the church to be put on the tree. Worst of all was the confusion of collecting children and presents for the trip home.

All this, my father reasoned, was done just to make a big showing; the practice so disgusted him that it spoiled Christmas giving for him. On Christmas Eve we hung up our stockings, and received a few inexpensive and homemade presents, although I have known him to rush downtown while we were at the church program, to buy a few last minute gifts. On Christmas Day we had a dinner such as only Mother could prepare, ending with pie, plump and juicy with her homemade mince. On the whole, our Christmas celebrations as a family were happy, even though sensible—and at home.

In our church, as in most Methodist churches of the early days, the preachers were changed almost every year. For one year we had the Reverend Mr. Brown as a pastor. His only child was a boy named Guy, who was just my age, eleven. Even the Ladies' Aid could find no flaw in this well-mannered lad, with big brown eyes and dark hair that just naturally stayed combed. He would hold his head on one side and look at you with a shy, wistful smile, as if he hoped you would like him. And I did! I fell in love with Guy Brown the first time I saw him!

That was the year of Charley's long bout with rheumatic fever. The parsonage was about a block away, and Guy came often to visit with him and to play quiet games. I usually managed to be on hand, but Guy gave no sign that he was aware of my presence. I even tried to reach him by petting Buddy, the pug dog with wrinkled face and twisted tail that shadowed him, but Buddy just looked at me with watery eyes, turned his snub nose higher, and walked away.

That winter the big boys tried to make a skating pond in the school yard, pumping and carrying the water by hand. Then the townsmen brought the hand-operated fire engine to help, and we had a skating pond.

One day I went there to skate, after school because I was just a beginner, and the pond would not be crowded then. Probably for the same reason, Guy Brown was there. A few older girls had come to practice fancy steps. They teased Guy and followed him around, trying to get him to tell who his girl was. He wouldn't answer—just pressed his lips together so tight his dimples were great wells in his cheeks.

I tried to stay close to hear if he answered, but I couldn't keep up with them. Suddenly Guy wheeled and coasted near me, then slowed down long enough to whisper two beautiful words in my ear: "It's you!"

When I recovered from my surprise, I called to him, hoping to get him to come back and say it so the big girls would hear, but he hurried to the other side of the pond, took off his skates, and started for home, Buddy at his heels. Now skating lost all interest for me. Skates flopping from a strap over my shoulder, I hippety-hopped home. Life was exciting! Life was beautiful! I was Guy Brown's girl!

And so, being more or less engaged to him, naturally I was worried when Mr. Brown came on a run one day while we were eating dinner and said Guy was terribly sick.

"What seems to be the trouble?" Father asked, as he shoved back from the table and went for his hat and medicine case.

"I don't know," the preacher said. "He didn't come when we called him for dinner, so I went to look for him and found him behind the barn, white as a ghost. He was so sick he couldn't tell me what was wrong." The two men hurried away.

Guy was sick! I had such a lump in my throat that I couldn't swallow, so I left the table, ran upstairs and threw myself on the bed. "He mustn't die! Oh, God! Don't let him die!" I sobbed.

Later, when I heard Papa come home, I slipped down the enclosed stairway and listened, knowing he'd probably tell Mother about Guy. I heard him say, "Some of the bigger boys got him to smoke a cigar."

How terrible! Tobacco was poisonous, especially for children —I knew that very well. Guy might be dying this very minute! I crept back up the stairs and threw myself on the bed and sobbed.

Father must have heard my weeping. He came up to my room and lifted me to my feet. I threw myself into his arms and begged, "Oh, Papa, don't let Guy die. He was wicked to smoke, and if he dies now he might—he might—" It was too horible to say.

He put his arm around me and said, "You mustn't worry about Guy."

"But, Papa," I insisted, "I'm his girl. He told me so. I'm his best girl. How can I help worrying?"

Now he pulled me close to him and I buried my face against his shoulder. I couldn't see his face, and he didn't answer for a minute, then he said, "My dear child, Guy isn't going to die. He's feeling better already. And you needn't worry about his smoking any more. He told his father he was sorry, and I'm sure that by now he's realized what a foolish thing it was to do."

I was reassured to some extent. Guy would probably not want to smoke again, and I resolved that, wicked or not, I'd love him forever, for I was his best girl. He'd told me so!

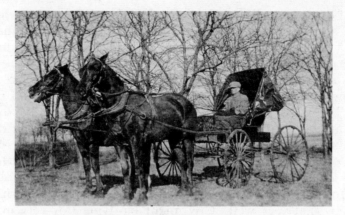

A strong team and a sturdy buggy were of
vital importance to the country doctor.
With them he faced all roads and weather.

Chapter 7

HORSE AND BUGGY DOCTOR

I REMEMBER hearing Father tell about his first horse, a spirited
youngster named Billy. Before we children were on hand to
make his acquaintance, Billy had been disposed of, and for
a good reason. It seems that previously he had belonged to a
young fellow who tried to make a racehorse out of him and failed,
but succeeded in spoiling him for anything else. Father was unaware of this history when he acquired him on an account, but
he soon learned that Billy felt compelled to race anything that
came alongside him.

Father preferred to jog along at a moderate pace, unless he
was on a hurry call, and often someone tried to pass him. Now
this was Billy's signal to race, and he was off before Father could
pull in the slack of his lines; but after a few near runaways he
learned to keep a tight rein, and for a while had less trouble.

However, one morning he started up a road that followed the
railroad for half a mile, then swung across the track. A train was
just pulling away from the station and they passed it easily, then

drove slowly to give the train time to clear the crossing. Father held Billy back, with some difficulty, as the train gained speed and caught up with them. Just at that moment it whistled for the crossing. Startled, possibly taking it for a dare, Billy bolted up the road. While Father pulled frantically on the lines and even sawed the horse's mouth with the bit, the young rascal dashed across the track, ahead of the train by so small a margin that Father (so he said) felt the engineer's breath on the back of his neck. Then, with Billy under control, he pulled off to the side of the road to quiet his nerves and to decide on the quickest way to get rid of a horse that just wasn't suitable for a young doctor to drive.

We had other horses in the early years, but I remember best Jim and Baldy, the team he drove when, as a child, I sat proud and happy beside him and rode with him over the countryside. Now Jim and Baldy were not the perfectly matched bays one sometimes reads about. Old Jim was a heavy chestnut roan with a small white star in his forehead, while Baldy was a smaller, raw-boned sorrel; his name was suggested by a white strip that ran from above his eyes back over his head.

But though poorly matched in size and appearance, the two pulled together beautifully. Sometimes I checked on this as we drove along; I'd lean over the dashboard to look at the whiffle-trees and I always found them in a straight line.

Those horses understood Father and knew when they could loaf along; too, they felt their responsibility when he was on a confinement case. The stork traveled fast in those days, but given half a chance old Jim and Baldy could beat him every time.

Then there was the old buggy. I don't know how long Father had it. I think this was his second, but I can remember only the one. When I hear of an old country doctor who wore out three or four buggies in a lifetime I know he didn't have a man like Sam Law to take care of them. Sam was our village smith, mighty and honest as the one immortalized by Longfellow. He used to nurse the buggy along, much as Father nursed the four little Laws through everything from plain stomachache to diphtheria.

Even when some intricate part of the mechanism was broken, Sam could usually make a replacement. Carrying the white-hot metal from forge to anvil he hammered, bent, and shaped it to his liking; and Father was spared not only a long wait for parts from the factory, but unnecessary expense as well. Sam once remarked, "You know, Doc, so many parts of that old four-wheeler have been replaced, I figure the only thing left of your original buggy is the hole the axle pin goes through."

And, of course, in addition to repairing the buggy, Sam kept the horses shod. This was fascinating for us children. We'd watch him shape a shoe to fit, and wonder how the horse could stand so patiently while Sam lifted each foot in turn and nailed a shoe firmly to the hoof.

An even greater attraction was the blue-flaming forge with sparks sailing high. When as a little girl Edna ran away, Mother usually found her standing spellbound in the doorway of the blacksmith shop. She used to say she was "watching Sam fix Papa's buggy," and often he was doing just that.

Now Sam may have been right about the "original buggy," but as I think back it seems to me that there must have been something else about Father's rig that remained unchanged all those years—a certain individuality made up of sound or vibration, a squeak not touched by grease, or possibly the clack of the feet of two proud horses who timed their steps to compensate for their difference in size. Whatever it was, Father's patients in the country recognized the sound as soon as he came within hearing.

And this was good, for many times as he drove along the road on a call, a housewife ran out and frantically waved her apron to signal him to stop. Maybe the baby was running a fever or Grandma's heart was acting up, and she was really worried; still she hesitated to call a man in from the field to go for the doctor. At such times it seemed providential to have him appear.

Now of course a "way call" cost less than a trip all the distance from town, and sometimes a householder took advantage of this, particularly when he knew Father would be coming by to see a patient farther down the road. But a greater nuisance was the man who would hail him only to say, "Hello, Doc! Just thought I'd stop you to find out who's sick down the line."

Both situations were alleviated when rural telephones were installed—I believed they appeared about 1904. Then news spread more quickly, and Father was spared many trips and still could keep in closer touch with his patients. And even greater changes resulted a decade later when automobiles began to come into general use by country doctors. But Father never owned a car. Even with Sam Law to look after it Father would have had a hard time to keep up a car, for he was not mechanically gifted.

But after all, what could be more pleasant than to jog along a country road behind cherished animals who returned one's affection, with time to listen to a meadow lark's song; to see a carpet of spring flowers or the satiny ripples of a field of new grain; or to watch young colts kick up their heels in a clover pasture? On pleasant days we could fold back the top of the buggy, and we really had a convertible, 1900 model, two horse-power. Waterproof curtains with isinglass windows and slots for the lines enclosed it against a storm.

There was a compartment on the back of the buggy that one might call a trunk, which held the two medicine cases. One was the brown leather satchel that, as well-informed children knew, brought the new babies. When I was very small I once took a peek, goaded by the curiosity of neighbor children, but it must have been off-season for there was no baby there.

A few years later I could have identified some of the contents: forceps for difficult deliveries, sponge forceps, splints, cotton, and rolls of homemade bandages. Then there would be a large piece of rubber sheeting; for this the early doctor found many uses. It could be spread to protect a table or bed during minor surgery, or to protect a patient under unsanitary conditions—even on a dirt road or in a barnyard where there had been an accident. It proved an excellent tourniquet, or a temporary cast for a broken limb. Less versatile but quite important was a pair of white muslin obstetrical pants to be worn by a woman during delivery. This and the generous use of boiled water and homemade soap were among the doctor's best weapons against childbed fever.

Just as important was the black, boxlike case with its neat rows of small bottles, for Father had to carry and dispense medicine in the rural areas. He must always have with him such drugs as calomel, quinine, acetanilide, ipecac, arnica, ichthyol, paregoric, digitalis, belladonna, bichloride of mercury, spirits of ammonia, and various tinctures.

Some medicines had appeared in tablet form as early as 1872, but they were not in general use, and capsules were unknown. Father carried a spatula and mixed and measured powders, which he wrapped in individual doses each in a small paper with the ends neatly tucked in; and he did it with such deftness and speed that it was fascinating to watch him. He left the patient an equal number of thin square wafers. One could be laid on a teaspoon and moistened in a glass of water; then the powder was put in the center, the corners folded over it, and with a sip of water it could be swallowed so easily that even quinine disappeared without a trace of the taste.

You can see that, from a utilitarian viewpont, the horse and buggy were well suited to the demands of the times—and to the roads. If, looking from your glassed-in, heated car, the old buggy still seems cold and drafty, consider Father's fur coat, his fleece-lined mittens and cap, the heated bricks and soapstones, the heavy blankets, and sometimes snuggled underneath but used with caution, a lighted kerosene lantern.

When I went with him I was dressed warmly too, with heavy wool dress and jacket and mittens. And long underwear! Not snug knitted ones, but homemade underpants of gray buffalo flannel, cut long and straight and roomy enough to allow for two years' growth! Oh, the tears I have shed as I sat on the floor and tried to crease those bulky drawer legs so they wouldn't look bumpy under my black ribbed stockings! I remember dressing on winter mornings as about the most unhappy experience of my childhood. I envied Edna who seemed to have less trouble, but as I look back now I think possibly she just couldn't be worried about lumpy stockings. The horrid garment was designed to keep us warm, and it did that; but is it any wonder that we always begged (in vain of course, for our health-minded father always said to wait until June) to be allowed to shed our long underwear the first warm day of spring?

Like other little girls of the Iowa nineties, I always wore something on my head; in winter it was a flannel-lined red velvet bonnet tied under my chin, sometimes with a long scarf wound around head and face so that only my eyes peeped out. In summer I usually wore a practical sunbonnet made of straw matting with blue calico crown and ruffle. I always yearned for a white sunbonnet with embroidered ruffles; but, though ever so fancy, a sunbonnet would still not be proper for Sunday best, and Mother rightly felt she had plenty to do without laundering a white sunbonnet for everyday wear.

Despite the weather, work went right on for the doctor. Father was prepared for even the wind and driving rains of late fall after Sam Law, working with his specifications, made for him a closed-in, boxlike body with a rounded top, mounted on two wheels, and similar to the old horse-drawn milk cart. Gloomy-looking to begin with, it was painted a dull black, and Sam named it the "Black Maria." It usually stood in the backyard, and we children found that between trips it made an excellent play house.

Although it had a door in the back and a large window in front, I preferred going in and out through the small windows in the sides, probably because it was one of the few things I could do that Edna, being larger, couldn't. However I failed to keep in training, and to my sorrow I tried it once after too long a lapse of time, for I had gained several pounds in the wrong places.

On this occasion, when but halfway through the small window, I found myself stuck fast, one-half of me yelling and wildly clawing the air, the other half kicking and reaching for a toehold. The half that was exposed to the weather and to the jibes and slaps of my sister and my supposed friends wore (it being Sunday) a creation of white muslin with embroidered ruffles—but it wasn't a sunbonnet!

My cries and the laughter of the other children brought Mother and Father to the kitchen door. Although he laughed harder than anyone, Papa came to my rescue and between chuckles comforted and reassured me. Outside, Mother reached up to support my poor aching legs while Father sat down on the swivel seat inside and said, "Now, Carrie, put your arms around my neck and hold on tight. We'll get you out. Got to. Can't drive old Black Maria with you hanging through the window. Now we'll just ease a little pad of flesh right here; now on the other side. Now see if you can turn a little bit. That's fine!" He continued to talk as he worked and presently he said, "Now we'll both pull hard. A little more—and there you are, all in one piece. I'll bet you won't try that again." He rubbed my sore muscles and patted me before he went back, still chuckling, to the house. That day the Black Maria lost its appeal for me.

During the years that Father had the odd vehicle, it was a popular Halloween target for the frolicking youth of the town. Once they succeeded in getting it up on the roof of the schoolhouse, but there was no truth in the story they told another year, that they had got the doctor to the door in his nightshirt, hauled him in the Black Maria three miles into the country and left him there with no way of getting it, or himself, home.

However, Baldy and Jim once came near to accomplishing that feat. They resented having to pull the Black Maria and would run, shaking their heads in a vain effort to rid themselves of what apparently was to them a monstrosity. One time Father used it for a trip five miles into the country. While he was in the house with his patient the horses pawed and snorted and shook, until in some way they succeeded in getting untied. Then they started running and never stopped until they pulled into their own barn.

Much more to their liking was the graceful sleigh that glided over packed snow so smoothly that on a short run one horse alone could pull it, although both horses were needed to go a long distance or to fight wind and storm. Whenever possible I went along for a sleigh ride, and it seemed to me that Jim and Baldy enjoyed the ride just as much as I did. Possibly they too appreciated the musical tones of sleigh bells with the rhythmic accompaniment of horseshoes on hard snow and overtones made by steel runners cutting the icy crust. Music became a lullaby as my lungs filled with the sweet, cold air. Then Father would slide forward so I could stretch out on the seat behind him; I would bury my face in his fur coat and go to sleep. I still have a nostalgic love for the smell of fur.

But jogging along with sleigh, Black Maria, and buggy through all kinds of weather finally began to tell on the horses. First old Jim began to break, and when a suitable horse was found to replace him he was pensioned and put out to pasture on a farm east of town. Some time later I went with Father when he had a call out in that direction. As soon as we turned onto the road that led past Jim's pasture, Baldy picked up his ears and quickened his pace. He knew that road, and when about half a mile away he began to call, "He-he-he-he-he!" Soon there came an answer—and another—and presently we could see old Jim straining his neck against the nearest fence corner of his pasture. As we came near we left the road and drove over to the fence, and the two old cronies rubbed noses and talked in soft whinnies, while Baldy's new sidekick pawed the ground and switched his tail in disapproval.

Presently Father spoke to Baldy and we started up, driving alongside the fence while Jim followed inside to the end of the pasture. Then, back on the road, we drove slowly as long as the horses could hear each other call. As we hurried on I could see Father's eyes were moist. And when he went in to see his patient I threw my arms around Baldy's neck and cried.

For a time Baldy's new teammate was a beautiful dark bay with a white diamond-shaped spot on his forehead that gave him his name. When we found that Diamond could not hold up his share of the work, he was driven single for a while and another horse replaced him. As he grew older he became fat and lazy, and though we all loved him, he hardly earned his keep. Then a young widow, who said she needed a gentle horse to take her children for drives and to visit relatives in the country, seemed to offer a good place for Diamond's semiretirement and he was sold to her. That would have been fine had she not let the grocer's boy use him.

One day when Charley and I were downtown we saw the grocer's spring wagon piled high with groceries, while half a dozen big boys rode on the seat or stood behind it. They laughed and shouted, while poor Diamond strained every muscle to pull the load, and nearly fell in the slippery mud on the street. Charley ran toward the wagon. "You stop that!" he cried, shaking his fist at them, but the boys only shook the lines and, more thought-less than cruel, urged poor Diamond on. We ran home in tears to tell Papa.

We could see that he was angry, but he tried to calm us, then said, "Now don't you worry. I'm sure that will stop when the lady finds out—" He grabbed his hat, and before we could ask what she would find out or how, he was halfway down the block. We saw no more abuse of old Diamond.

Now with just one look at our next horse you could guess his name. He appeared to have more bones than usual for a horse, and most of them could be located at a glance. "Old Bones" was already named when Father acquired him in payment of a long-standing bill. Not only was he homely; he was exasperatingly slow as well, and, even worse, temperamental.

So much depended on Father's having good transportation that he soon gave up getting anywhere with Bones and gave him to Edna. Now fourteen years old, and with six years of music lessons behind her, she had a class of piano pupils scattered in the nearby countryside, and on Saturdays she drove out to give lessons. Bones seemed safe enough for her to drive, his worst fault being his inquiring mind. What would frighten many animals only whetted his curiosity and he would stand quite still in the road to look things over. If what he saw was a roadroller or a threshing machine, some man would probably come and, with a little per-suasion, lead the nag past by the bit so that both he and the young music teacher could proceed with their work.

If Bones heard voices in the buggy he stopped with ears

cocked for better listening. That wasn't so good one Saturday morning when Alice Lee and I went with Edna on her teaching trip. Out of respect for Bones' curiosity we had kept our voices fairly subdued until we got out on a lonely road, when Alice and I suddenly laughed out loud at something Edna had said. Old Bones stopped. We kept quiet until he started up again; then we all giggled, and of course he stopped again. After a few stops and starts we found ourselves laughing hysterically while Bones stood with feet firmly planted on the road, his head turned back as far as it would go, his ears pointed first back, then forward.

In a nearby field a farmer stopped his plow and stared at us, raised his big straw hat to scratch his head, wrapped his lines around the plowhandle, and started slowly toward us. Not caring to make explanations to a stranger, Edna used the buggy whip—harder than she had intended—and Bones gave a jackrabbit start that frightened us into silence for a while. Subdued, again we jogged along until Edna had given her lessons for the day; but she refused to drive Bones again, and he was sold to a farmer who, it was hoped, had less talking to do while driving.

After more than twenty years of hard country practice Father's general health, and particularly his hearing, began to show the strain, and he took a younger doctor in with him to relieve him of some of the long rides. When he did go into the country the family of the patient usually furnished the transportation, so that horses were not so necessary. Baldy had long since gone to join his old buddy, Jim, in heavenly pastures, and our only horse was a graceful bay named Nancy.

Charley was now in high school and Father tried to plan his calls so that the boy could drive Nancy when he had a date. On Sunday nights he would drive to the Congregational church and, at least for a time when the gods specially favored him, escort the pretty daughter of Father's old friend, the druggist, home by way of Lovers' Lane.

Now horseless carriages were making an appearance here and there over the country. Will and Glenn Schreiber, two of our high school boys with more than average mechanical ingenuity, mounted a gasoline engine on a sturdy, homemade chassis, and Sloan had its first automobile. So it happened on a certain Sunday night that the lovely Marie rode off in a gas-propelled buggy, and poor Charley drove Nancy home alone.

Next morning I happened to go out past the barn and

thought I heard muffled crying from the direction of Nancy's stall. All sympathy (I hope it wasn't mere curiosity) I stopped and listened. "Well, Nancy, old girl, it's all over." It was my brother's voice. Between sobs he went on, "I don't suppose I'll ever be so lucky again, Nancy. We did—did the best we could, d-didn't we old girl? And I'm not b-blaming you a bit. We just—just couldn't expect to beat an automobile."

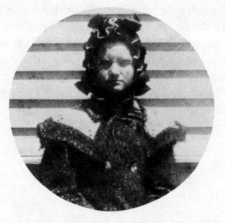

A flannel-lined red velvet bonnet helped keep Cora snug when she joined her father in making calls during Iowa's cold winters.

Chapter 8

A-CALLING WE WOULD GO

DURING Father's years in Sloan, a large part of his practice was in the surrounding rural area. Whenever it was possible, he took me with him on his calls in the country. I was always eager to go; I loved just being with him. Then too, he pointed out things of interest, and in many ways made the occasion pleasant and worthwhile.

The longer drives were a special treat—to places with such delightful names as Maple Landing, ten miles south of Sloan; Holly Springs, nestled in the hills ten or twelve miles to the northeast; and, five miles farther north, Climbing Hill. Given the transportation of the nineties, such a trip required about half a day.

Time spent with his patients varied of course. The usual consultation might last twenty minutes or more. But I am reminded of the time when, for many days, two-year-old Grace Montross hovered between life and death with a virulent fever. The children of his old friend George Montross were very dear to

Father, and his anxiety and the hours he spent with little Grace, day and night, continued until she was out of danger.

Probably the shortest call he ever made, both in distance and in time spent with the patient, was to the home of the Christian preacher who was our next door neighbor at the time. One evening, just as Father finished his supper, the preacher's daughter burst in the front door and called, "Doctor, come quick! Mother's choking on a fish bone!" Without wasting a second, Father picked up a roll of cotton; needing something to wrap it on to make a swab, he jerked the long coiled spring from the screen door and wound the end with cotton as he hurried down the walk.

As he neared the parsonage he heard the preacher praying, "O God, send help! Send the doctor before it's too late!" Hurrying through the door held open for him, he went directly to his patient, who was lying limp in a chair held tilted back by her husband. Her thin features were distorted, her face purple. With one quick motion Father picked up a small salt shaker from the table and placed it between her jaws, inserted the makeshift swab, and dislodged the bone. The air wheezed into her lungs; she sat up slowly, opened her eyes, and looked about her as though she had just arrived in an alien country. The preacher clasped Father's hand and said, "God bless you, Doctor Frear. Thank God, you didn't have far to come."

However, distance was not always so important a factor as the weather. One autumn day the doctor at Whiting asked Father to come down there for a consultation on a difficult case. The eight-mile trip would have been comparatively easy had not fall rains begun, making the roads sticky and deeply rutted. Rain still fell, driven by a cold, northwest wind.

Fortunately, or so it seemed, a train went down to Whiting about noon, and a freight was due for the return trip a few hours later, so Father decided to go by rail. He arrived at his destination in good time, and all would have been well, except that the conference took a little longer than he had counted on. Just as he ran puffing up to the station for the trip home, the freight started to pull away from the station. He could see that the caboose was too far down the track for him to catch it there, and that by the time it reached the place where he stood now, it would be going almost full speed.

Now Father had never climbed up the side of a freight car, but he had seen it done, and it looked easy; furthermore, the brakemen seemed to have no trouble walking the length of the train on top of the boxcars. There wasn't time for him to consider all the possibilities, so he just reached for the ladder, swung up, and climbed to the top of the car. He found that three narrow boards ran the length of the cartop to give better footing, but they were wet and slippery from the rain, which was still falling. Then too, the wind was stronger with the train heading into it.

Just as he reached the end of the first car, the train lurched suddenly and threw him sprawling, face down. He seized the wet boards with both hands; he raised his head to look across the open space to the next car, then estimated there were twenty spaces between him and the relative security of the caboose; he remembered that his legs were short, his experience nil, and he wisely decided to stay where he was, hang on to the boards, and pray.

The run to Sloan took less than half an hour, but it seemed hours to poor Father before the train began to slow down. As it neared the station a brakeman found him and helped him down, soaking wet, stiff and numb from the cold, hatless, much wiser, and willing to trust Jim and Baldy and the squeaky old buggy for transportation in the future.

Even with the transportation problem resolved, the doctor of the nineties often found another hurdle between him and his patient—sickroom visitors. I witnessed this one Sunday when I went with him on a five-mile drive, leaving just before noon. Evidently word had gotten around at the rural church that "Charley Jones had a real bad attack. Inflammation of the bowels. We must go and see Charley." And what better time than right after church—all dressed to go, horses hitched up, and no farm work to do since it was the Sabbath.

There were so many rigs around the Jones place that Father had trouble finding a place to tie his team. I went in the house with him. A tired looking, rawboned woman motioned me to a chair and said, "You go right on in the bedroom, Dr. Frear." Wearily, she added, "That is, if you can get in."

He made his way between women sitting stiffly in their closely buttoned black basques and full skirts, and a group of men, uncomfortable in celluloid collars. He spoke to some of them by name. Presently I heard his voice from the bedroom: "You stay here, Mrs. Jones. I'll need your help—but the rest of you please wait outside. I'll call if I need you." A man and a woman came

74

out angrily, stormed out of the house, and drove away. Two men followed sullenly and closed the bedroom door.

From where I sat beside the parlor door, I heard snatches of conversation, most of it in hoarse whispers:

". . . exactly like my cousin Andy, and he was dead in three days."

"He doesn't have any insurance. . . ."

". . . and undertakers cost something awful!"

A baby cried; its mother turned her chair away, unbuttoned her dress and put the child to her breast. The hushed talk continued.

"I told Amy to send for Grandma Shikes. She knows more than all the doctors put together."

"She'd use a dead chicken poultice. . . ."

"No, that's for gangrene. She'd slap a fresh cow manure poultice on his belly before you could say 'Jack Robinson.' Ain't nobody can make 'em like Grandma Shikes. She'd have him out of bed in no time."

Just then someone turned and saw me sitting there, eyes wide open, ears tuned in, and said, "Little pitchers got big ears." She got up and closed the door. So I turned to watch the kitchen lady. Her dress was wrinkled, her hair stringing in her face. She jabbed a hairpin in her knot as she went to fill the stove from the woodbox, then rubbed her eyes and left a smudge. Grabbing the water bucket, she filled it from the pump outside, poured the water into the dishpan and the teakettle on the stove, then sat down at the table spread with dirty dishes, and buried her head in her arms.

The fragrance of apple pies and hot slaw filled the kitchen; there were a few pieces of fried chicken in the skillet, and I was hungry. I was thinking she might ask us to eat dinner, when Father came out and she said, "Can I fix you some dinner now, Doctor?"

He looked at her and hesitated, then he looked at the work piled up in front of her, and said, "No, thank you, we'd better be going."

Tears came into her eyes and she said, "Thank God, there's one person with a heart. Doctor Frear, I have gotten dinner for twenty-three people here today."

In another home, there were no visitors to annoy the doctor, but the patient's children had proved a problem. One day I was to go with him, and as we were about to start he took an empty

75

bottle from his medicine case, scratched off the label, and filled it with cornstarch from the kitchen cupboard. As he worked, he chuckled to himself and whistled his funny little off-key tune.

"Is that medicine?" I asked.

"W-e-l-l, I hope it will cure something; we'll wait and see," he said. He wouldn't tell me more, though I asked a dozen questions, except to answer that the mother was sick, and yes, they had children, and no, he didn't think they would play with me. After a six-mile drive we turned off the road and followed a weedy lane for a quarter of a mile to a small run-down house. As we approached, an undetermined number of children poured out of the house—all small and so much alike with their sunburned hair and blue eyes that I wondered if there were several pairs of twins. At one time I counted eleven, but I couldn't be sure; they moved too fast as they swarmed around the horses and over the buggy.

They wanted to carry the medicine cases, but Father declined their offer and tried not to step on them as he went into the house. He took me into the kitchen and said, "You wait right here," as he pointed to a chair beside the table. It proved he had given me a ringside seat.

Two children tried to follow him upstairs, but a pleasant, dark-haired girl they called Kate pulled them back; she proved to be the hired girl. Despite her efforts to get them to go outdoors and play, they stood and stared at me or whispered and giggled. This went on until Father came downstairs, when the stares were turned on him.

And really, he did seem to be putting on a show. He opened his medicine case with a flourish, set several bottles in a row, and studied them carefully. He spread a sheet of white paper on the table. The eleven (by a second count) children crowded around to watch, shoving against him as they fought each other for position. When Kate tried to stop them he shook his head at her and I could see his eyes twinkle.

Now he selected two bottles, and with a spatula, took a generous amount of cornstarch from one, and a smaller amount of white powder from the other; he scraped and turned and mixed the two piles together seriously, his open-mouthed audience watching every stroke. They were breathless when he scored the mixture off into small squares. Then he took a generous pinch of the powder between his thumb and finger, put it in his mouth, smacked noisily, and licked his lips.

76

In a flash, eleven small hands reached out and eleven samples of the mixture popped almost simultaneously into eleven mouths. Then the storm broke! The youngsters howled, they spit, they coughed. They stampeded the waterbucket with its one dipper, then dashed for the pump. Kate laughed so hard she couldn't help them, and Father and I laughed with her; then, as the children disappeared, he went calmly about his work. He mixed, measured, and folded individual doses of powders into neat paper packages. It was fascinating to watch him, but the children were no longer interested.

After a few words of instruction, Father snapped his case shut, motioned to me, and we were on our way. Outside he paused to clear his throat and wipe out his mouth with his handkerchief. "That's a new use for quinine," he said as he got into the buggy. "I didn't get that from a medical textbook either, but, by the Georgetown Harry, I bet it'll cure them." From all reports the cure was permanent; he had no further trouble with those children.

Later that year I went on a trip with him that was entirely lacking in humor—in fact, it could have ended in tragedy for both of us. Father had an emergency call over in Nebraska, and ordinarily we would have crossed the Missouri by ferry—always a treat for me. The river was only about six miles from Sloan, but news travelled slowly in those days, and it was not until we arrived at the landing that we learned that the ferry was not running because the "Big Muddy" was too swift and rough. The spring thaw in Minnesota and the Dakotas had swollen the streams there, and hurrying south they had joined the river to build up the torrent that we now watched from the shore—the worst June rise in many years.

The river was not over its banks but was cutting badly. The sloping wooded shore on the Nebraska side withstood the beating, but when the current swung to the Iowa side, it pounded and slapped at the steep bank, six or eight feet below the ground level, until strips of land a hundred or more feet long and three or four precious corn rows wide toppled over into the swirling water.

On this day the ferry landing was deserted except for a stocky, bronzed man who sat stripped to the waist, bare feet dangling over the water, and fished. His skin was tough and wrinkled, his eyes squinted from sun and reflection from the water; his arms were deeply scarred from sunburns of previous summers, and his arm and shoulder muscles bulged from straining at the oars. John Troth had been born and raised on these banks and his whole life was tied in with the river. To eke out what subsistence the river and a small garden plot gave him, he sometimes sold fish in town, and often rowed a cargo or a passenger across the river. John was now Father's only hope of reaching his patient.

Father called to him, "How's the fishing, John?"

"Ain't much good. Too swift," John answered as he reeled in his line and ambled over to where we stood. Father explained his errand. John looked out over the water and hesitated. "She's pretty rough, Doc."

"And you're a good man with a boat," Father said.

"Yeah, I've crossed her when she was a heap sight worse," he said proudly. "But knowing her like I do, I gotta respect her. She'd carry us downstream if she didn't pull us under."

"We can walk back up on the Nebraska side."

"Kid go too? They get scared and rock the boat."

"She goes where I go. She'll not bother you." He mentioned what he would pay, and it looked pretty big to John.

His eyes measured the opposite bank and he looked up- and downstream before replying. "All right. Boat's up here a piece." We followed about a hundred yards upstream to a place on the bank where a flat-bottomed rowboat was tied to a tree. John got in, then Father handed me down and followed. He sat beside me with his arm around me, my hand in his. As we pushed off and felt the first impact of the current, my heart missed a beat and I buried my face in Father's coat. But at that moment he called my attention to some boys fishing on the western bank. We tipped and rolled at first, and at times a wave splashed over us, then the boat yielded to John's handling as if it were a part of his body, and I became more calm; as I watched him my confidence increased. Now he gave a little, now he fought the force that tried to turn the boat and pull it downstream.

The water was so muddy that it was a dull tan in color. Branches and small trees and boards floated on the surface; a chicken house, tilted crazily, headed toward us while a dozen Plymouth Rock hens flattened out on the roof or clung precariously to the edge and cackled or squawked out their fear. John remarked, "Someone down the line'll get a free chicken dinner," as he swung right to miss them, then reached out with an oar to ward off a section of a fence.

Once we were beyond the current, we reached the Nebraska shore without any further trouble. John beached the boat and said he'd take a nap while we were gone. As we started to follow a path up the sloping bank a man hailed us from above. He had watched us cross the river and was waiting with a buggy to take us to our destination. He was a neighbor, he said, and while he and Father talked I tried to imagine to what sort of a place we were going. I knew only that the patient was a little girl about two years old. They were probably rich people, I thought, since they could send clear to Sloan, in a different state, for a doctor (although probably there was no doctor closer). I was sure they had a lovely home and many toys for the child.

Just then the neighbor said, "Here we are," and stopped beside a run-down, one-room shack. There was no door—an old quilt covered the doorway, and broken shingles were nailed where windowpanes were missing. Inside, a stove, a table, a bed, and a few chairs comprised the furnishings. A young man sat on a box in the corner of the room, his head in his hands. On two chairs spread with a folded comforter and placed in the warmth of the cookstove lay a small, very quiet child, her eyes half-closed. One little hand clutched what looked like a pillowcase rolled to make a doll, its features marked with ink on a face scarcely whiter than that of the little patient.

The mother hovered over her baby, watching Father's face anxiously as he made the examination. I, too, studied his face, then I slipped outdoors—I didn't want anyone to see me cry. I sat on a stump and looked out over the river until Father came out. In answer to the neighbor's question he said, "I think she will recover, but she is a very sick little girl."

We found John asleep on the bank, looking as peaceful as though the Missouri River were a gentle, babbling brook.

The wind had gone down, the current seemed less angry, and John headed upstream. Then we saw the tree to which the boat had been tied topple into the water. He swore and turned sharply to find a low place where we might land. Soon it was all over, and the welcome ground under our feet gave us a feeling of security as we walked back to the buggy. We got in, Father clucked to the horses, and our adventure was over.

Father was quiet for a while, then he said, "A kind Providence seems to have watched over us today. I think I'll show my appreciation by doing a good deed. I'll go by and see the Millers."

In answer to my questions he explained, "The Millers used to be good patients of mine, even before I left Salix. They farmed, and did pretty well while the boys were home; but they're alone now, except for her sister Mandy. They worked too hard—they're old before their time—so now they have pretty hard sledding."

"Are they sick, Papa?"

"Not that I know of. Never sick much, just old and run down. It's hard for them to get in to the office, so I stop in and see them now and then. Keep them supplied with tonics, physics, things like that, and maybe a little advice. I haven't sent them a bill in years. Glad to do it for them. Nice old couple."

A little later we reached the Miller place, the common type of story-and-a-half, L-shaped farmhouse; it needed paint, but the yard was raked clean and flowers bordered the short path.

Red-mustached Bill Miller's greeting boomed from the porch, echoed by Molly's reedy, "Come right on in!" They led us through the kitchen with newspaper-covered walls, freshly laundered sash curtains, and green woodwork and wainscoting, soft-soap clean. I saw that the table was set for supper and, to protect it from the flies, covered by a square of cheesecloth feather-stitched in red. Fresh-baked bread cooled on a rack.

The "settin' room" still held a cheerful look although its rose-patterned wallpaper and rag carpet were faded. The large family Bible shared the center table with a red plush album, a mail order catalogue, and an empty salmon can that Bill used for an ash tray. Molly motioned me to a seat on the sofa and brought me a cooky, then handed me a stereoscope and a box of the two-view photographs.

She sat in a high-back rocker, prim and unsmiling, her white hair drawn back so smooth that it reflected the colors of the patch-work velvet of the antimacassar. Her liver-spotted hands twitched nervously on the chair arms.

"That your oldest?" Bill asked, indicating me with his pipe stem. "Second, eh? You don't say! How time flies!"

"She's the one who usually looks after me on my calls in the country. We just went through quite an experience," Father said, and told about the river trip.

"Was John sober?" Bill asked with a grin.

"Dead sober, today. But drunk or sober, I'd trust old John with a boat farther than anyone else I know."

"That's right. Best river man around here," Bill said.

There was an awkward pause, then Father asked, "Well, how have you been?"

"Pretty good—we can't complain," both answered quickly. The air of restraint grew heavier.

"And Mandy? Is Mandy all right?" Father looked from one to the other. Molly's restless fingers creased and smoothed out folds in her apron.

"Well, no, she ain't," Molly answered hesitantly. "Mandy was took awful sick a week ago. She was awful sick, Doctor."

"Where is she?" Father seemed puzzled by their obvious embarrassment. When they didn't answer at once he went on, "She didn't—don't tell me that Mandy——"

"Oh no, she ain't dead. No, not that. She's still in bed, though," Molly answered while the old man watched her closely and pulled hard on his pipe.

"Well, I'll take a look at her. But why didn't you call me? You know I'd be glad to come any time," Father told them. "If you can't pay it's all right. You should know that by now."

"Oh, we know you would," Molly said quickly. "You've been awful good to us, Doctor Frear. But you see—well—" she stammered, and looked appealingly at her husband.

Bill took it up. "You see, it was like this, Doc." He emptied his pipe with three sharp clicks on the salmon can and put it in his pocket. "Mandy was took so sudden, and she was awful sick. She was so sick we thought we'd better have a *pay* doctor this time, so we sent to Salix for Doc Taylor."

Father chuckled over the incident as we drove home, and in later years often told it as a good joke on himself.

I shared many pleasant drives and interesting experiences with Father that summer when I was ten, and when school started I missed them. Evidently Father missed me too. There was a morning when I came home from Sunday school to find the team hitched up with Father waiting for me to eat the quick lunch Mother had set out, and join him on a trip "over in the hills." He didn't even ask if I wanted to go; he knew and shared with me my love for the low-lying hills east of Sloan, and for the prairie we must cross in the ten-mile drive to reach them.

I ate quickly, pulled on the warm coat Mother held for me— it was cool riding in late September—and tied my red velvet hood as I ran to the buggy. Father tucked the lap robe around my knees, slapped the horses' backs with the lines, called "giddap," and we were on our way.

As we drove through the north part of town with the buggy top down, I waved to some of my schoolmates, feeling sure they envied me this nice Sunday drive. Then we turned east. There was little of interest in this level, sparsely settled country. The few farmhouses were as a rule rough, unpainted, and small compared to the red barns, machine sheds, and corncribs grouped behind them. There was always a windmill; sometimes a few maples or box elders had been planted for shade and a windbreak.

We talked as we jogged along, mostly about my new teacher and school problems. When I told him I didn't like "jogerphy," he casually told me about some of the places he had seen in this country, and others he would like to see. Then he hinted that someday I might even travel all over the world, and see some of the wonderful countries I was studying about; I could hardly wait to get back to my desk and the big, new textbook that had seemed so difficult.

Presently the conversation lagged and Father was half-humming, half-singing, in his funny way:

> Oh, why should the spirit of mortal be proud?
> Like a fast-flitting meteor, a fast-flying cloud. . . .

Only now, as usual, the words sounded more like: Da-de-dum, da de dum, de da-da-de-dum.

All this time we were on one of the rough dirt roads that divided the country into mile-square sections. The soil here was fertile and, under favorable conditions, produced abundant crops; but after heavy rains, it became a sticky gumbo that defied cultivation sometimes for an entire season; on the roads it rolled up on the wheels, so that a driver was obliged to carry a shovel and stop occasionally to scrape off the mud so he could proceed. But today the road was dry, with hard, deep ruts which, once they were in them, the wheels were obliged to follow.

After a few miles we reached the edge of the prairie. We could cross it diagonally to save a few miles, so now we turned off the dirt road. This was always exciting, even frightening, for drainage ditches edged the road and the banks were steep. The horses stepped down cautiously, pulling back against the harness; there was one brief moment when the rear right wheel poised in the air, then it settled down as the team began the hard pull up the other bank. I held on tight and pretended I wasn't afraid; we never had tipped over, and we didn't this time. We were safe on the wide prairie. Here we followed a wagon trail—two deep ruts made by wheels and hoofs, with grass growing between them—which cut in a northeasterly direction across the prairie. Neither of us spoke—that would have seemed irreverent—and above the rattle of the buggy and the plop, plop of the horses' feet we could hear the swish of the tall grasses that surrounded us.

Although I had often crossed the prairie, each time the sense of space, the loneliness, and the beauty surprised and delighted me anew. I even loved the name—"prairie" had such a mysterious sound, and it purled off my tongue as if a part of the grasses that rippled in the breeze or, at times, dipped and rose again like ocean waves, following one after another as far as the eye could see. To-day the grass, taller in many places than a man, was shaded in color from tawny yellow to bronze, while the deep blue sky covered it like an inverted bowl.

Near the trail a cottonwood tree clacked its thick, shiny leaves together, reminding us that it alone of all the trees had survived the drought of past summers. The sumac flaunted its autumn leaves for an occasional splash of red on the yellow sea. A compass plant, tallest of the prairie weeds, pointed its leaves north and south. Sunflowers hung their once proud heads, their yellow crowns now withered.

A covey of prairie chickens rose from beside the trail with a whirr of wings; a bobwhite whistled, "M-o-r-e wet!" Father laughed and said, "All right, boy, we can use some rain."

We made our way leisurely until we were about halfway across the prairie, when we noticed that the horses seemed in a hurry. Heads forward, ears back, they pulled ahead. "The wind is coming up. The horses feel it," Father said. Just then a jackrabbit coming from the west leaped across the road, so close to Jim's feet that he shied, startling Baldy. A plover flew over our heads with a frightened cry. Father tightened the reins as the horses shook their bridles and pulled on their bits.

Now more birds flew overhead, more rabbits and smaller animals scurried past us. I wondered if they were being chased, and pulled myself up to look back over the buggy top. I probably expected to see some huge wild animal, but for the moment the landscape failed to show anything unusual. Then I looked farther to the northwest, and cried excitedly, "Oh, Papa! Look at the funny clouds!" But he was having trouble with the team.

I looked again, and now I could see a red glow in the sky. Suddenly I remembered a story of a prairie fire in our school reader, and I knew what those rolling clouds meant. "Papa, it's a fire! Look quick!" I cried, and he turned to look.

"Oh, No!" he moaned.

Realizing our danger, I started to cry. "What'll we do, Papa? We'll be burned up!"

"No," he said quietly. "No, I don't think so. Don't be frightened." He didn't sound too reassuring, but after all he was my father and he had always taken care of me, so I waited, and watched him, quiet, almost afraid to breathe.

Now he had the horses under control and he pulled them to the left, and windward, side of the trail. "Raise the buggy top, and bring that blanket from the trunk," he said to me as he got out, tossed the lines over the horses' heads, spoke to them soothingly, then looked about. It was evident that we were too far from any exit from the prairie to escape, but looking to the southeast, he said, "I think this will do it."

I was beside him as he made a little pile of dry grass and fumbled in his pockets for a match. He didn't smoke, but he sometimes carried matches to light the lantern when he needed one at night, and he had a piece of one now. He knelt, and with a hand that shook a little, he struck it on the sole of his shoe. It didn't light and I knew from the look of despair on his face that it was his only match.

Instantly I was off for the buggy, calling, "Your old vest!" I had seen it in the trunk when I got the blanket. I was back with it in seconds, and in the pocket we found one, only one, match. As he struck it I leaned over him and spread my skirt as a shield. There was a tiny flame, a crackling sound, then flames leaped into the air as he pulled me back to safety.

The blaze fanned out in front of us, racing and leaping with the wind. We were conscious of the peril bearing down upon us from the northwest, but there was no time to look back, for Father was using the blanket to beat back the flames that crept along the edge of the trail, and I used the old vest to help him. Since the wind was in our favor, we were able to keep the fire from crossing the trail, so Jim and Baldy and the buggy were safe for the present. Father spoke often to the horses and they stood, restless but obedient. Finally, when the newly burned area had cooled sufficiently, we got in the buggy and drove out over the charred remains of our beloved prairie.

I choked back a sob, then, remembering that we were safe for the present at least, I whispered over and over, "Thank you, God."

When the dense smoke closed in around us we stopped and left the buggy to stand between the horses, holding the blanket so as to cover their heads and ours. Now the flames, their path split by our burned area, raced to the right and to the left of us; heavy smoke rolled overhead nearly choking us, and the heat was terrific. But we were unharmed, and after a few minutes, we were able to emerge from our makeshift shelter; we shook the blanket, brushed a few bits of burning debris from the buggy top, and got in to resume our trip. When I saw Father had headed the team northeast again, I begged, "Can't we go home now?"

"No, my dear child, we may be needed more than ever now," he said, "possibly by someone living along the path of the fire. These farmers protect their buildings with firebreaks—they plow strips around them and burn the grass between them—so probably the homes and the people are safe, but even so it is a terrible experience." I could understand that, after what we had been through.

We rode in silence for a while, then I said, "Papa, I prayed while you struck that last match."

"I'm glad you did," he said. "That match saved our lives."

As I turned to look at him, a drop of perspiration ran down his face, leaving a clean streak that looked like a crack in his blackened cheek. I laughed out loud and he looked at me, and I suppose I was as black as he was. He laughed and said, "We'll stop at the Addison's—that's the first house we come to—and get washed up. I could use a drink of water too."

As we turned in their lane, Mrs. Addison came running out and cried, "Oh, Dr. Frear! The good Lord himself must have sent you! Tom's terribly sick."

Father found that the man had suffered a mild heart attack when the fire threatened their place. Fortunately he could take care of the condition and assure them that Tom was in no immediate danger. A little later we left, refreshed by cookies and milk—and a shade cleaner.

We were hailed as we passed the next farmhouse, where the man of the house had been badly burned in fighting the fire when it jumped the break. At another house a woman's fright had brought on hysteria and severe indigestion. But at last we reached the creek where the fire had stopped, and as we crossed the bridge and left the blackened prairie behind us, the hills seemed to welcome us with a cool, clean embrace.

Soon we reached the home of the patient who had originally sent for Father, and eventually we started for home.

As we approached the prairie I tried not to look at it. Then I saw that he intended to cross it. "Do we have to go back this way? Anyway, how will you ever find the road?" I asked.

"The horses will see to that. They brought me across this prairie once when it was a solid white, instead of black. It was night too, and all I could see in every direction was snow."

"I guess the angels must have led the horses that night."

"I believe you are right. It must have been angels," he said and was quiet. I pressed him to tell me more about it, but he said, "Ask your mother sometime. She'll tell you about it."

All this time something had been troubling me. I dreaded to hear the answer, still I just had to know, so I whispered, "Papa, will the prairie ever be the same again? Will it come back?"

He nodded. "It will all come back. We'll drive out next spring, and you'll see the green grass and flowers——"

I interrupted, "The bird's-foot violets? And the pinks and the Indian apples?"

"That's right. And later the long grasses and the sunflowers; and the prairie chickens and the bobwhites. They'll all be here."

Relieved, I laid my head on his lap and soon I was asleep. When we crossed over to the dirt road again, I woke up and looked around. The blue bowl overhead had changed to indigo, a fitting background for the stars that were appearing.

When we were about a mile from town Father pulled the horses to a stop and said, "Hark!" But I was already listening. The three bells from the three churches announced that it was time for the evening services. Each had its own tone and timing, still they held to a rhythmic musical pattern, and like the individualists they called to worship, at intervals all joined in one harmonious chord.

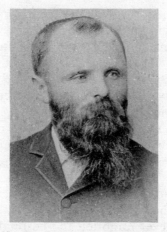

By 1895, Dr. Frear's hair was beginning to thin. But, like many substantial citizens of the day, he sported an impressive beard.

Chapter 9

DOWN IN THE BEND

ABOUT five miles southwest of Sloan the Missouri River made a sharp turn to the west, then curved back to a point about five miles south of the turn. Some of the richest bottomland in Iowa lay in this area—the number of acres would depend on when the survey was made, since the Big Muddy changed its course, cutting corners here and there, seemingly at will. The farming country here and spreading to the east was usually referred to as "the Bend," or, more specifically, "the Norwegian Bend," since most of the residents were sons of Norway, or their descendants, the others being Swedish, Danish, or American.

The town of Albaton was the trading center, with a post office in J. Polly's general store. Although the population was only about thirty, there were two churches, one Methodist, one Lutheran, with a cemetery spread out between and beyond them.

Shortly after the 1900 census had been taken, Father, having made a call nearby, stopped in the store to get some coffee; he claimed the Norwegians demanded, and got, the best coffee that could be bought. Someone mentioned the census; Father remarked that they had been shortchanged. "How's that?" he was asked.

"They didn't count everybody," he said, motioning toward the graveyard. "Why, there are more than twice that many people between here and the church!"

Immediately a sandy-haired, blue-eyed man, sitting with a group around the stove, spoke up: "Da's right, Doctor Frear, and you is yoost de one ought to know. You done more'n anybody else to fill dat place up."

Father had a nostalgic as well as a practical interest in the community, for he had taught school here during his first year in Iowa, and he had never forgotten the hospitality and kindness of the Norwegian people.

In this school, only one of the seventeen pupils, a boy of eight, could speak English; he acted as interpreter, and Father gave the others lessons in the English language, along with their sums and letters.

More than sixty years later, Horace Bakke, who, as a boy of seven, had attended the school at the time, told us that he had sprained his ankle during the term, and would have missed school if Father had not called for him and carried him pickaback both ways, every day for a week.

Returning to the community six years later as a physician, Father had watched these children grow to adulthood, marry, and become established on their own farms; he had delivered their babies and cared for their sick. These young people and their parents, friends of the early years, became a large and loyal part of his practice.

Also in this neighborhood he had experienced many of his professional "firsts." At one time he was called to see a man who was in terrible pain which centered in a swelling on his right side. It was evident that here was an abscess, and that immediate drainage was necessary. They were thirty miles from a hospital, and there was no time to waste. Father made the incision, unassisted. The relief was only temporary—the disease had progressed too far. It was not until a few years later that he learned he had performed an operation for appendicitis, basing his conclusions on a report of nine case histories of appendicitis, given by Dr. Will Mayo before the Minnesota State Medical Society in 1888.

In 1896 Albaton and vicinity had an epidemic of diphtheria, with an alarming number of deaths. When twelve-year-old Reuben Hunter showed early symptoms, he became Father's first case to receive antitoxin treatment. Speaking of the incident some forty years later, Mr. Hunter said, "I remember that my back was stiff all summer, but at least I didn't die like a lot of others did." He recalled that Dr. Huff of Onawa, fifteen miles south of Sloan, had used antitoxin previously. (It was first placed in the hands of the general practitioner about 1895.)

It was understandable that Father enjoyed his work down in the Bend. His contacts with the Norwegian people had always been congenial; he admired their honesty, diligence, and loyalty, and thoroughly enjoyed their sense of humor. He was interested in their background and culture too and liked to take us children with him into their homes. I, even more than Edna or Charley, was always ready to go. I liked the ride, but I liked more to see treasures they had brought from Norway, such as pictures, kitchen tools and dishes, and lovely handwork.

I remember especially one call we made, when I was quite small, on a family recently come from the old country. When about a mile from our destination, I saw some bright buttercups and asked Papa to stop so I could pick some. He said, "Wait till we come back. We'll have more time." He always said that, and usually came back another way. But this time he glanced at his watch, studied it a minute, then clucked to the horses and hurried them along.

He seemed in such a hurry that I asked, "Is someone awful sick, Papa?"

"No, not that I know of," he answered.

"Then why are you in such a hurry?"

"You wait and see," was all the explanation I could get. He urged Jim and Baldy on, looked at his watch again when we were nearly there, tickled the horses with the buggy whip, and minutes later we dashed into the yard of a big white house at breakneck speed. He stopped with a jerk and said, "Jump out quick and run into the house. Don't stop to knock. Hurry!"

Obediently, I started on a run. Someone saw me coming and opened the door; as I stepped inside the room, my attention was drawn to a whirring sound coming from the wall in front of me. There hung a funny little clock shaped like a house, its hands pointing to twelve, and before my unbelieving eyes a little bird hopped through a tiny door and whistled, "Cuckoo!" not once, but twelve times!

When I had recovered from my surprise, I heard Father laughing behind me. "Now do you see why I was in such a hurry?" he asked. While he took care of his patient, her daughters kept me supplied with cookies and milk, and when we left I carried gifts of fruit and handwork for Mother from the grandmother.

With a patriotism that should put some of their American friends to shame, these newer citizens turned out on the Fourth of July, usually with a big neighborhood picnic, to celebrate their independence. Much of the food was prepared in large quantities by several women working together. The days preceding the celebration were busy ones for the housewives; sometimes the days following were equally busy for the doctor.

One year, calls started coming in the early morning hours of July fifth, and as he hurried along the road, Father was hailed and asked to see others who were ill, often several in one house. People of all ages were afflicted, some seriously, others less so, and the symptoms in all cases were the same—severe vomiting and diarrhea. It seemed that one thing all the patients had eaten was potato salad which had been made by the dishpan full. The trouble was not too hard to trace; with no refrigeration available, the hard-boiled eggs had not cooled sufficiently before being added to the salad, and ptomaine had resulted.

Again on a July fifth Father was called to many of the same homes, but this time only women and children were affected. The men thought this was a good joke. "It vas beer dat cured us," they said. "Ve tol' you beer is goot for us."

Father said maybe they had a point there and followed it up. What did the women and children drink? It proved to be lemonade—and that would have been all to the good, except that it had been made in a copper boiler!

Another year there was a real epidemic. Perhaps this one followed the union picnic of the Bakke and Gullickson schools, rather than the Fourth of July, but at least fifteen families attended. A few days later Father was called to see teen-aged Herbert Gullickson. He was not seriously ill and, according to the report, had no intention of being examined by the doctor, so he hid in the barn. The embarrassed parents finally produced the patient, who insisted there was nothing wrong with him; but he could not hide an eruption of shot-like papules which was unmistakably due to smallpox. Of course he had attended the picnic, so no one was surprised when dozens of cases broke out in the community.

Now Father had no fear of smallpox (as we shall see later) and for about a week he made a daily "smallpox trip," looking after all the patients. Most cases were light; one exception was the husky-looking Anderson boy, in his late teens, who continued to work in the harvest field even after his temperature rose to 104°. After he finally gave in and went to bed, he was critically ill for two weeks. Since practically everyone in the neighborhood was exposed at once, and all cooperated in the strict quarantine imposed, there was no spreading of the disease, and no serious results of the epidemic were noted.

Though not planned that way, all being ill at once seemed consistent with their way of life, for family togetherness was very strong among the Norwegian people. In the homeland the entire family would plan to seek a new home and broader opportunities in America. First, all would contribute to send two of the young folk across. These two would work hard and save to send for two more. With four working, soon others followed; eventually the whole family would be brought to their new country.

Father watched as this plan was worked out in a family of eleven children. The first two soon were able to send for two more, then three others joined them. The industry and loyalty of these seven young people impressed Father and he rejoiced with them when they were able to send for the rest of the family: the parents, their three teenagers, and the oldest son with his wife and three small children. The day they were to arrive Father went to the train, and while he remained in the background he enjoyed witnessing the reunion.

He liked the appearance of the old father, Adolph Haanestedt, a small wiry man with a stubby beard and twinkling blue eyes. After he had had two weeks to visit with his children and see something of his new country, Father went to see him and, through an interpreter, offered him a job caring for the horses and garden.

The old man thought it was some kind of joke and refused to consider the proposition until relatives who knew Father convinced him that the doctor really wanted him. So in the end he came, very humble and ill at ease because he was unfamiliar with the language or customs of the country and did not know what would be expected of him.

He nearly wept with embarrassment when we insisted that he eat at the table with us, but Father put his arm across his shoulders and almost forcibly led him to the table. There he ate little and soon got up, made a prim little bow, and said *"Tak för Mäten"* as he left the table. After a few days he accepted the arrangement and relaxed a little, but the first chance he had to speak through an interpreter he told us, "I cannot write to my friends in Norway that I work for an American doctor and eat at the table with the family, for they would accuse me of telling lies about my new country."

Father tried to recall some of the Norwegian language he had picked up while teaching in Albaton, and Mr. Haanestedt persevered in trying to learn English. Whether we broke a dish, shelled peas, or put out the cat, he would ask, "Vat calla du datta?" Then, his eyes twinkling, he would repeat it over and over and ask, "Iss goot?" By the end of two weeks we could communicate, if not converse, with him.

Adolph Haanestedt stayed with us until frost ended the garden work, when he joined his family, and with them planned to become part of the farming community in the Bend.

Soon after he left we had in our home another man from that area, one whom I shall always remember. Edna and I were in high school and becoming interested in parties, when Father announced one day, "Tomorrow I'll bring Olaf Johnson down from the hospital, and he will stay with us for a week before going on home."

Immediately we girls objected loudly. "But we have planned to have some of the girls in for supper Sunday night."

"Then he will make one more guest," Father answered with an emphatic nod. Edna suggested weakly that he could be fed ahead of time. "There is no distinction here between guests," we were told, "we all eat together."

Then something clicked in my mind. "Who is this Olaf Johnson?" I asked, hoarse with apprehension. "Isn't he the one they call 'Dirty-shirt' Johnson?" We girls did not know him, but we had heard the name.

"The name is *Mister* Olaf Johnson," Father insisted.

We turned to Mother for help. She only laughed. Dirty-shirt Johnson it was, and there was no appeal. We called off the party.

With uneasy curiosity we awaited his arrival. We saw a small, shy man with a soft voice. He wore a black sateen shirt, but it was immaculate; that was the first thing we noticed. Then we looked at his face; his forehead was high, his eyes wide set and intelligent; his dark hair was rather long, after many weeks of illness, and curled a little about his neck and ears; his mouth was sensitive and sweet, and there was a spiritual beauty about him that reminded us of pictures of Jesus.

He was quiet and unobtrusive, and most of the time he sat in the dining room and read his Bible. He wouldn't come into the parlor; but one day Edna played the Norwegian national hymn, and he came to stand in the doorway and listen, with a faraway look, his eyes filled with tears. "It is beautiful!" he whispered. We coaxed him to sing it for us; he finally yielded and we found he had a sweet tenor voice.

He said he loved music. Once he had heard Ole Bull, the great Norwegian violinist, give a concert. He tried to describe it to us. "At first the music seemed to come from up above us, then from far away. Then it was everywhere around us. It was—so sweet—" He hesitated, seeking words to express himself.

We learned he had heard the violinist in Christiania while he was a student at the university there. Gradually he warmed to our genuine interest and told us something of his early life. He had been left an orphan at the age of nine and was to make his home with an uncle who lived sixty miles away; he walked the entire distance alone, over the snowy mountain passes of Norway. Later, he planned to prepare for the ministry and had begun his studies. Having to make his own expenses, he worked nights as bookkeeper for a store; but that, added to his college work, had proved too hard on his eyes, for he had gone temporarily blind and was obliged to abandon his plans for an education.

While still a young man, he had come to America to make his way, first working on a farm, where he met and married a girl from Norway. They had started to farm on their own. It had been a struggle for one who was not built for heavy work, but he had succeeded, as we learned later; too, we heard from time to time of his grandchildren, who carried off scholastic honors that had been denied him.

For us, "Dirty-shirt" Johnson ceased to exist as we grew to love *Mister* Olaf Johnson. Through knowing him, we began to understand some of the truths Father had tried to instill in us: the error of snap judgment, the equality of man, the beauty of humility. We were reminded of the words of St. Paul: Be not forgetful to entertain strangers, for thereby some have entertained angels unawares.

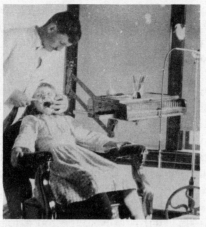

Handsome Uncle Charley practiced his dental technique on Cora. A foot-operated pedal provided the power to run the drill.

Chapter 10

OFFICE ASSISTANT IN PIGTAILS

I DON'T REMEMBER when I chloroformed *my* first patient, or vulcanized the first set of dentures, but I know I was an old hand at both when I was twelve years old. I might be called on at any time, back there in Iowa before the turn of the century. Father's younger brother, Charley, or Nick as we usually called him, now practiced dentistry and shared Father's office. He had been with us ever since our return from Pennsylvania, when he was eighteen and I was four years old.

At one time Father had considered sending his brother to medical school, so, to give him a taste of a doctor's life, he took him on calls with him and enlisted his help in many practical ways. Possibly his choice of contacts with a country practice was ill advised. For one thing, he sent the young man to collect some long-standing bills in a poor farming country.

Nick returned with no money, an old hen, a small pig (the runt of a litter of eleven), and a bushel of wormy apples. An

Indian from whom Father expected nothing more than a gruff "Ugh!" gave Nick a load of wood, which followed him home. His pride in this deal fell when he learned that the wood (which Father said was slippery elm) had a high degree of immunity to both ax and fire.

Then one winter night Father was called to the scene of an accident. He knew he would need help in handling patients and making splints, so he called his brother. Under protest, Nick got out of bed to go with him. It was only six miles, but the temperature was thirty-eight degrees below zero. They arrived home just before dawn, unharmed, but the experience cooled any enthusiasm my Uncle Charley may have had left for the practice of medicine.

However, his skill with tools suggested a logical compromise, and he enrolled in the University of Iowa to study dentistry. Now he was back; Father made room for him in the office. He also shared his office girl; I was their combined receptionist, dental technician, doctor's assistant, errand girl, and janitor, serving part time and without pay. My uniform was a blue print dress, or maybe the brown gingham one, whichever I had worn to school, with black ribbed stockings and high-buttoned shoes. So my Uncle Charley, who would have loved having a pretty technician in a crisp white uniform working beside him, had to settle for plain little me, in calico and pigtails.

In spite of my tender age and inexperience, he was really good at finding things for me to do. I washed the instruments and dried them carefully so they wouldn't rust. Asepsis was still in the experimental stage in the hospitals. I had never heard of it. His drills were run by a foot pedal that he could perfectly well operate himself, but he convinced me that I could do it better; sometimes I held a lamp, or a mirror to reflect the light from the hanging lamp or window, so he could see into the patient's mouth. To set an inlay he held a blunt instrument against it, and I tapped the other end with a light wooden hammer.

Among less specialized tasks, I cleaned the spittoon and spread a newspaper on the floor to set it on. I fastened fresh towels to the headrest of the red plush chair, filled the waterbucket from the pump out back, occasionally washed the dipper, and swept or mopped the oilcloth which covered the floor.

What I liked best was taking care of children while their mothers were having work done, but this was mere play compared with serving as an anaesthetist. When a patient put up a fight while having an extraction, Father might have to help hold him as well as watch pulse and breathing—in fact sometimes a man off the street was also called in to help. In such a case, I was often drafted to hold the gauze-covered mask over the patient's nose and pour the chloroform drop by drop, always under Father's watchful eye, while he checked the patient's reaction and nodded directions to me. (At this time ether was replacing chloroform, but because of its flammable nature, it was unsafe to use where the operator depended on open flame for light, as was the case in Sloan.)

While thus "professionally" employed, I heard so many people make so many kinds of fools of themselves while "coming out from under" that I vowed never so long as I lived would I submit to an anaesthetic. I remember one old man whose droopy mustache kept getting in the way during the extraction. He was an exhorter for some religious sect, and as he began to wake up he sang hymns and prayed for Father at the top of his lungs. People over on Main Street heard the noise and hurried over, curious at first, then they stayed to laugh at Father's embarrassment after they learned what was happening.

Women patients whined and complained of their housework, then yelled loudly for the children to "Hustle a basket of cobs for this fire," or "Git them chores done in a hurry." One woman started to air her views on men in general, and her husband in particular, but I didn't get to hear much of what she said, for Father suddenly decided they didn't need me any more and sent me to the house on some trumped-up excuse.

But the patients who impressed me most were the girls—old and young—who made love to Uncle Charley. Although modest and timid in their conscious moments, scarcely presuming to raise their eyes before him, they became bold as they emerged from their unnatural sleep and asked for his ring, a date, or a kiss, or insisted on holding his hand.

You couldn't blame them, for Uncle Charley was the real "flaming youth of the gay nineties." His gray eyes were deep set under long, curling lashes and his wavy, blue-black hair, parted on the left side, dipped low on his forehead, then swept sharply back in a long, soft curl. His chin was square and manly, and his mustache—ah, there was a mustache! Black and crisp and ending in smartly curled tips!

As if that were not enough, he knew all the popular songs, including: "Just Tell Them That You Saw Me," "She Was Happy Till She Met You," and "The Baggage Coach Ahead"; and he sang them in a pleasing tenor voice, accompanying himself on either the banjo or guitar. Because of his talents and ready wit, he was in demand anytime, day or night, when young folks got together, and I'm sure it wasn't his fault if his social life sometimes interfered with his practice.

No doubt I should have been thrilled to do things for him. Maybe I would have been but for the "torture chamber." This was a room about five by seven feet with built-in worktable and shelves, which he fondly called the "laboratory." Since I spent as little time there as possible, I can't say what all was "labbed" therein, but I remember supplies of various kinds, many of which had to do with making false teeth. (I wouldn't have known what dentures were.) Also, there were usually a number of plaster-of-Paris models on the shelf—not figurines, but impressions of some unfortunate oldster's jaws; and having seen these molds made many times, and having watched the patient gag on the wet plaster-of-Paris packed in a metal form, I made a second resolution—that never, never would I have false teeth.

Now dental plates had to be vulcanized, and if I didn't find out about it in time to get away I was, too often to suit me, elected to watch the vulcanizer. This was a small pressure chamber heated over a small kerosene stove that sat on the laboratory workbench. It was called the "S. S. White Vulcanizer," but the "S. S." did not stand for Sunday school, I decided, and white was definitely not its color after a few sessions with that smoky oil stove. It could have been a man's name, of course, but why he should want his name on such an ugly contraption, I couldn't understand.

Anyway, we turned the stove wick up or down to regulate the temperature. To start with, it took at least half an hour to reach the required 320 degrees, and it had to be kept there for an hour and twenty minutes in order to maintain the proper pressure to "set" the teeth in the plate.

I remember that the first time Uncle Charley left me alone to watch it he warned me that if I let the pressure get too high the vulcanizer would explode and blow up the laboratory and me with it. Of course it might explode anyway, I was told, as he left me to my fate.

So there I sat on a high stool in that stuffy room with the

window closed to keep drafts off the stove. There were fumes from the burning oil mixed with the odor of oil of cloves and carbolic acid and iodoform and cigar butts and bloody towels soaking in a bucket of water. All this time, my eyes were glued to the thermometer except when I dared steal a glance at his watch hung on a nail beside the window. Perspiration streamed down my face and hair got in my eyes unheeded, for I knew that to relax for one moment might mean death to me—and someone's false teeth ruined in the bargain.

Of course I might be blown up anyway, I remembered, but martyrlike I stuck to my job. I wondered if Uncle Charley would weep over my charred remains, and what the *Sloan Star* would say about me. Then, after an eternity, the time was up and I turned off the stove with a vague sense of disappointment that nothing had happened. My name wouldn't be in the paper after all and no one would know how brave I had been. Uncle Charley would give me a nickel and forget the whole thing—or more likely, forget before he gave me the nickel.

I got even with him once though. He asked me to watch the office, saying he was going out, without saying where. He had worked out a very clever system whereby he didn't tell me where he was going—he wrote on a piece of paper where he could be found and laid it in the instrument drawer. Then if one of his buddies or a very special patient came in I could consult the paper and locate him quickly; otherwise, I truthfully could say I didn't know where he was.

On this day a Mr. Brown came in, a man who always wore a collar and tie, so to my eleven-year-old way of thinking he was a rich man, hence a very special patient. While I consulted the slip of paper to see where my uncle was, I naively explained the system to Mr. Brown, thinking he would feel flattered to be considered "special." He was interested, very much, and even asked a few questions, which, unfortunately, I answered as fully and truthfully as possible. Then I offered to go and get my Uncle Charley, but Mr. Brown thanked me and said, "I guess I won't need to see him after all."

Uncle Charley never could understand why Mr. Brown suddenly quit coming to him just when he had planned to have some bridge work and two inlays made, and had his dental work done in Sioux City. I offered no explanation because I didn't know—for sure.

99

Now it was inevitable that so popular a young man as this uncle of mine would get married. I remember the night in November, 1898, when we rode out a mile or so east of town to the home of Myrtle Bird, the lovely bride, for the ceremony. It was clear and cold, and showers of falling stars made a display that was beautiful but a little frightening to us children. Years later we learned that we had witnessed an unusually brilliant shower of Leonid meteors.

Soon after their marriage the young couple moved to Kansas. Later, another dentist, Dr. Charles Lacy, came to share the office. He was a quiet, dignified man in his early twenties, and since he also had a room in our house for many years, he became an important member of our household. Because his training had been more modern, and he had by nature a practical, orderly turn of mind, his influence led Father to see a more modern and practical approach to some office problems. While Dr. Lacy never intruded, he was just enough older than we children were to understand us and to interpret our notions and ambitions to our parents, and at times to advise us and give us a more cooperative viewpoint. But Dr. Lacy—I never heard him called "Charley" except by his sisters—seemed to be quite able, in fact, preferred, to do his own vulcanizing and to care for his own instruments, and that suited me fine.

I still spent much time in the office but I was just Father's helper. Besides doing office errands I waited on him while he dressed wounds, but I suspect that he invented things for me to do so as to keep me there beside him. My specialty was still the care of young children who came to the office with their parents. One day when Father sent for me to come to the office I found there a young couple from over in the hills fourteen miles east, and with them their twin baby girls, who were about ten months old. Imagine how thrilled I was! I had never taken care of twins, and I wondered if I could rock two babies to sleep at once. Then Father explained why he had sent for me. It seemed I had outgrown baby-tending—I was all of eleven—and my professional services were needed. I was to put one of the babies to sleep, but with chloroform, so that he could remove a black birthmark about the size of a penny from her cheek near the lobe of her ear.

She was a dainty child, smaller than her twin, and her bright, dark eyes followed us about and watched without fear as we prepared for the simple operation. In later years I watched Father remove such blemishes with a carbon-dioxide pencil—dry ice to most of us—but surgery was probably the only remedy in use at the time. He explained to the parents that there would be a scar, but that it would not be disfiguring and that it would show less as the child grew older. It did not occur to me at the time that someday I would verify his statement.

About four years later—I was fifteen at the time—a different sort of case came from the same neighborhood. A five-year-old boy, towheaded Albert Ralston, had a broken collarbone. This happened to be the third fracture of the same sort to be brought in within a few weeks. When the first came, Father called me in to watch him set it, explaining each step as he did so. The second one came soon afterward, and he had me set this one while he watched and gave advice.

Just at the time that the Ralstons brought little Albert in, Father was starting out on a confinement case where trouble had developed. The Ralstons had seven children and knew only too well how serious a delay at such a time could be. Accordingly, Father took time only to examine the break, and when he found it was similar to the one I had set recently, he told the Ralstons that I could set it as well as he could, and they had such confidence in him that they took his word for it. After a few instructions to me he hurried to the waiting buggy and the case was mine.

First I padded the lid of a talcum can to give pressure directly over the break; then I held it firmly in place while I started with a long bandage, which I crossed and recrossed at this point as I carried it over and around his shoulders in a figure eight. I told Albert it must be as tight as possible without hurting him, but to tell me if it was too tight. His blue eyes never left my face, though they filled with tears and his lips quivered, but he only shook his head when I asked him if it was too tight. I remember that I lay awake half the night thinking, with a sympathetic constriction in my own chest, of stoical little Albert and wondering whether he could breathe.

Five years later, when I had finished college, Mr. Ralston asked me to teach the one-room school of which he was director, so in September I found myself facing twenty-two children, most of whom were strangers to me. They ranged in age from five to seventeen, from beginner to seventh grade, and I had had neither experience nor training as a teacher.

On the first day of school most of the boys wore new overalls and had fresh haircuts, and their faces had been scrubbed until their freckles had a polished look. I recognized Albert Ralston, now ten years old, his blond hair still standing straight up from a cowlick on the left side, his blue eyes as frank and steady as ever. At the first recess he came up to show me how well his collarbone had healed, and he was as proud as I was when I had difficulty in finding where the break had been.

While Albert and the other boys looked their freckled best, the girls were sweet in their first-day finery of starched calico and polished high-buttoned shoes with patent leather tips. Bright hair ribbons fastened long braids, or framed the pink-cheeked faces of the smaller girls whose hair hung loose. Many a busy mother had taken time the night before to wind her little girl's hair up on rags to make curls or had plaited it tightly so it would hang in pretty waves when unbraided.

There were four little sisters from one family—the Moulin girls. The smallest one, Eva, was especially attractive and I was conscious of her dark eyes as they followed me about the room, and of her winsome smile. For some reason, a scar on her cheek attracted my attention, although it was small and inconspicuous. I learned that she and Ava were twins although they were not alike in size or appearance. A few days later I was invited to the Moulins' for dinner. Mrs. Moulin asked me, "Do you remember the first time you saw the twins?"

Surprised, I asked, "Why, have I seen them before?" Only when she reminded me did I recognize Eva as the baby from whose face Father had removed a birthmark while I assisted with the anaesthetic.

But to leave the schoolroom and go back to the office: I remember so well a day when I was thirteen. Two tall girls in their late teens brought their two-year-old brother to the office. His right leg was swollen to twice its normal size and he made little whimpering sounds as if too weak to cry aloud. Examination proved he had an abscess which had to be lanced at once and I was called in to assist with the anaesthetic. Meanwhile the sisters, who had come to help the doctor, helped only by keeping out of the way. They walked up and down the boardwalk, weeping and wringing their hands.

I remember how easy it was to put the little fellow to sleep; since there was no fear of the anaesthetic to overcome, with each fluttery sob he drew the pungent vapor into his lungs. It was only minutes until Father could begin the operation, which proved most disagreeable because the infection was so far advanced.

I kept one eye on the baby's respiration as I stood beside Father ready to follow his every suggestion. I dodged the spurt of pus from the first incision, then tried to catch and wipe up the discharge as he pressed and probed the swelling. When the worst was over I suddenly realized that Father had stopped his work. Looking up at him, I found his eyes on me, with an odd expression on his face. I studied him for a moment, wondering if I had made some mistake, but there was no criticism in his look. Neither of us spoke, but messages flashed between us. "Am I doing all right?" my eyes questioned, and his kindly look answered that I was doing fine, so I was content.

But there was something more in that look that I did not understand at the time. To me there was nothing unusual about a thirteen-year-old child who faced, without flinching, a sight that might well have sickened a professional nurse. I accepted as a matter of course my presence there beside him, for I always wanted to be where he was, so I just grinned up at him, and he smiled back at me and gave his funny little chuckle as we both went back to work.

We had paused only a few seconds, but in that time the look on my father's face was in some way impressed on my memory. I can recall it as though it were only yesterday, and I believe that I know something of what it meant to him to have me working there beside him. I believe it was for him then, as it became for me later, one of the beautiful experiences of life.

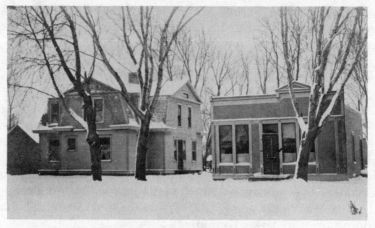

The Frears were proud of the new house the doctor had planned and built. His office was moved beside it from a downtown lot.

Chapter 11

THE NEW HOUSE

FOR MANY YEARS Father and Mother dreamed, planned, and worked to have a permanent home, a comfortable house large enough to accommodate not only the family, but also the relatives and friends who always seemed to be a part of the household. They started building during the autumn of 1898, but the work progressed slowly—with money scarce that year—even after the lots were bought and the plans drawn up by a Sioux City architect. Since Father was determined not to go in debt for the house, most of the work was done "on account" and he had to wait until the men could sandwich his work in between more remunerative jobs. We moved in before walls and woodwork were quite finished.

He refused to hire contract labor, feeling sure that the construction would be slighted, and he personally knew enough about carpentry—having worked at it in his twenties—to oversee the work and even to direct and instruct some unskilled workers.

They did not always agree with his methods; they objected to using twice as many nails as was customary; they grumbled at the weight of the native cottonwood sheathing which covered the house diagonally before the siding was put on; the men couldn't see the sense of putting plaster on the sheathing when he'd have two coats over the laths on the inside wall.

But Father was determined to have a well-insulated house. At first he talked of building a house that would withstand a cyclone, but he said no more about it after a few old-timers had expressed themselves on the subject; those Iowans had great respect for their cyclones; still it was a well-built house.

To get sand for the plaster, Father engaged Joe Sloan, a farmer east of town, to haul two loads from Sand Hill Lake, about seven miles from Sloan. I remember it well, for Joe's daughters, Bertha and Fannie, were my best friends; Joe drove one team, Bertha drove the other, and Fannie and I rode with her. It was a warm October Saturday, and we took a picnic dinner. Then, while Joe took his time to fill the two wagons, we three girls played in the sand and loafed through a hazy, lazy, never-to-be-forgotten day.

I remember too the time that Father's personal interest in the details of the work nearly ended in disaster. The "drove well" was in general use in Sloan at that time, and the water was hard and unpleasant in taste. Father planned to have a "dug well," the sides to be walled part way down with bricks. One afternoon when the well was nearly finished, and after the men had gone for the day, he decided to inspect the brickwork. He asked Wilford Pirtle, a big redheaded high school boy who did our chores for his room and board, to let him down a little way into the well with the windlass. It was like Father to forget that he was wearing a new linen suit. He had been lowered a few feet and was examining the wall when Wilford's hand slipped from the windlass, and poor Father dropped into the well with a sickening splash. The men had struck yellow clay and water had begun to seep in, so that there was about a foot and a half of sticky yellow mud in the well.

Wilford looked down and saw that Father was safe, but spattered clear to his head, coughing and spitting as he tried to wipe the mud from his eyes and mouth. The boy saw only the funny side of the situation, and without so much as an apology he started to laugh—not a polite snicker, but one uninhibited guffaw after another. This stirred up seldom-tapped depths of my father's vocabulary, and that only made it funnier to Wilford, so that it was several minutes before he could control himself enough to operate the windlass, pull the poor man to the surface, and help him out. Then Father waddled home across lots, dripping with indignation and gobs of juicy clay.

Wilford sat on a pile of lumber and laughed for a while, then went home expecting to share the fun with the family, but it wasn't funny to Mother. The doctor was safe, but she couldn't forget how serious the accident might have been—and she still had to launder that linen suit.

Father had already taken a lot of good-natured ridicule about the surface water some said he would have to drink; now, as the story of his immersion spread, his "contaminated well" became the joke of the town. However, a few weeks later, when the well had been cleaned out and had filled with water, one had only to try it to be convinced that we had the best drinking water in town. It was clear, tasteless, and almost ice-cold, and on a hot day many people came to refresh themselves.

After we moved in, sometimes a rough-looking stranger would turn in from the street, go directly to the pump and drink his fill, then leave without so much as a look at the house. One mid-day in July, Mother answered a knock at the back door to find there a tall, dusty man with a pleasant smile and a young face beneath dark, tousled hair. He lifted his hat, bowed, and said, "Ma'am, I've looked forward all morning to a drink from your well, and someone has taken the dipper away. Would it be asking too much—? Oh, thank you kindly, Ma'am!" With another bow, he accepted the glass she offered and came to return it ten minutes and a few pints later.

"I don't think I know you," Mother said. "Do you live in Sloan?"

"No Ma'am," he said with a smile; "I live wherever I can find a piece of dry ground or a pile of hay to sleep on and not get chased off. Last night it was in a barn somewhere the other side of Whiting."

"Then how did you know about our well?"

He laughed. "Why, Ma'am, I been comin' here even before your house was finished. Every tramp in the Missouri Valley knows he can get a good, cold drink of water here, and stops by every chance he gets. We are all very grateful, Ma'am, and I do thank you for your trouble." With another bow, he was gone.

So the Frear house had become a landmark even before we moved in! We were close to the center of town, and on the main road to the fairgrounds. On days when there was a carnival or ball game, a steady stream of people passed by; so many stopped for a drink that on a hot day our pump handle would go up and down for hours without stopping.

The office had been moved from its downtown location to the corner of our lot, so that it was about twenty-five feet from the house. We had a wide frontage on the street, and outside the boardwalk friendly maples spread their arms to cover the entire length, while others shaded the back of the lot. On special days families from the country were quick to take advantage of such perfect picnic spots, and our quiet corner came alive.

Father joined the picnickers whenever he could. He seldom saw these people when they were not sick; now he could visit and joke with them, as he did when a long-legged Frenchman from north of town strode by en route to a ball game. Father called out, "Hey, Louie, why didn't you bring your wife and kids along?"

Without stopping, Louie shot back, "There's too blamed many of them, Doc; you ought to know that."

Indians from reservations in Nebraska still made occasional visits to Sloan. One day three wagonloads of Winnebagos pitched camp in front of the house. Plump squaws with black braids and bright beads swung the tiniest papooses, strapped to their cradle boards, from the lower branches of the trees. Toddlers watched us solemnly from behind their mothers' long full skirts when we tried to coax them to come to us by offering candy or bits of ribbon and pretty pictures.

After dinner the squaws sold gooseberries which grew wild over in Nebraska. They went from house to house with a flour sack full of berries over one shoulder and a bright-eyed papoose held by a shawl peeking over the other. They spoke no English, but a quart measure and the five spread fingers of one hand indicated the price. On this day, Father found two old friends in the camp, Abe and Charley Wolf—tall, fine-looking Winnebagos whom he had known for years. He took me out to meet them, and visiting with two real Indians gave me quite a thrill.

Having the office near the house had a more practical side, too, for Father could call from the side door of the office for someone to help with a patient, look after children, or just bring a drink of water; it was easier, too, to find him when dinner was ready.

When he had a few minutes to spare, he would come to the house; always, as he opened the door, he called, "Sue? Oh, Sue!" If there was no answer he would start through the house, calling again and again, "Sue? Oh, Sue! Where are you?" and an alarmed note would creep into his voice.

Maybe she would run in from the garden and ask anxiously, "What is it, Doctor?"

"Oh, nothing, nothing," he would answer with undisguised relief. "I just wondered where you were." She would return to her work with no sign of impatience; she seemed to understand his need of her and to appreciate his devotion. It was her job, and her pride, always to be there when wanted.

Of course it was Mother who most enjoyed the new house with its added space and ample closets. There were eight rooms and two halls, and another room included for a large bathroom, but no plumbing was installed in the house while we lived there— not even a kitchen sink or running water. We did have a fine hot-water furnace, although we usually had to burn wood instead of coal. The insulation Father had insisted on had paid off, for the house was easy to heat in winter and was cool in summer.

We had many windows, and Mother especially enjoyed the large bay window in the dining room, which in the winter came alive with coleus, geraniums, and chrysanthemums—prim white, ragged yellow, and little red button mums that bloomed by the hundreds in her homemade window boxes.

Three years after we moved, Sloan installed a local telephone exchange. In these days when telephones are taken for granted, it is hard to realize what that could mean to a doctor at the beginning of the twentieth century, especially when it was shortly followed by rural lines.

To go back several years, the first telephone had been installed in Sloan about the time the folks moved there, in 1886. This was a long-distance line, and while at first it extended no further south than Sloan, it was possible to talk to Sioux City, and from there to connect with most large and many smaller places in the country. The first day, service was free from Sloan to Sioux City, and many residents enjoyed their first telephone conversations. Thereafter one paid twenty cents to talk to Sioux City, and twenty-five cents anywhere else in the state.

But it was not until 1903 that Sloan had its own telephone exchange. Working with the installers was a local boy only fourteen years old who, when the crude seventy-two line system was completed, took on the job of maintenance man for the year until he entered college in 1905. Whether the project was the result or only the beginning of his interest in telephones, his work was done efficiently, and his townsmen were not surprised when, forty years later, he had become nationally known as Dr. Oliver E. Buckley, President of the Bell Telephone Company's Research Laboratories; in 1951 he was made Chairman of the Board.

This early system was not complicated. We turned a pointer to the desired number on a dial and rang our party direct by turning a crank. When more telephones were needed, we acquired a "hello girl."

When Father learned that some of his clients had put in a telephone line connecting eight or ten families south of town, he realized what a help it would be in keeping in touch with his patients, and he suggested that they run their line into our house so that he could talk with them. As an inducement he told them (possibly without consulting the local owners) that he would connect them with the town phones. The farmers lost no time in carrying out this plan.

Then complications set in. Another neighborhood, then another, put in rural lines and asked for the same privilege. Before Father could work out a solution, there were ten or twelve lines coming in to a switchboard in our kitchen.

Then the owners of the town exchange decided that the rural patrons were getting too much free service and refused to let us connect them with the town phones. For a time we took rural calls and repeated the messages through our own phone. We tried not to order a blade for a scythe when one was needed for a mower, or mix the prices being quoted for wheat and for potatoes, but it all took time.

Soon we had one hundred twenty-five patrons on the rural exchange, and answering all their calls, plus messages to and from the town folks, had become a real problem. But Father, never dreaming there would be so many lines, had promised free service for a year. Now the farmers said that the lines had cost so much that they must economize for the present, but if we would hold out to the end of the first year, from that time on they would pay twenty-five cents a month for each patron. The Sloan businessmen demanded that connections with the farmers be restored, so that was taken care of. A new long-distance line asked us to take their calls. The work altogether was not too demanding, so we agreed to continue as central until satisfactory arrangements could be made for the rural exchange.

Mother took most of the calls on the farmers' lines and loved it. She took an interest in the patrons and their problems, which were many and varied. A tired young mother might call in, "Mrs. Frear, if anyone wants me in the next hour or so, please don't ring me. Just tell 'em the baby's better, and I'm trying to get some sleep." Or in another vein, "Mrs. Frear, Jim's in town, and if he tries to get me, tell him I'm out chasin' pigs, and if he knows what's good for him, he'd better bring something to fix that fence."

She could understand isolated farm women who listened in to get the news—that was the accepted pattern for neighborliness. But lifting the receiver while she was trying to ring weakened the line so that calls would not go through. By little things like a clock ticking near the phone, or maybe a canary, she learned to identify the patrons, and called by name, the offender would hang up.

On one line she often heard a rooster crow while she was trying to ring someone. Then one day a woman who seldom called in asked for a party. Just then Mother heard the familiar crow.

"Is that your rooster?" she asked. The woman laughed. "Yes, that pest! He hangs around the kitchen door all the time."

"Yes, I know," Mother said. "I often hear him when I try to ring on this line. Now, after this, please wait until my party answers, then you may take the receiver down and listen to your heart's content." She had no further trouble on that line.

Inevitably, the telephone business soon outgrew the corner of our kitchen. We were relieved when a company was formed to establish all phone systems in one downtown office. But once in a while a farm woman would call in to say, "We sure miss you, Mrs. Frear."

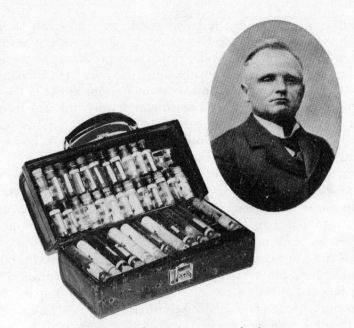

As the twentieth century neared, changes appeared in medical supplies and in the doctor himself. He shaved off his beard!

Chapter 12

QUARANTINE IN THE NINETIES

IN MANY DETAILS the house Father built had been planned with a practical, and also charitable, purpose in mind. Because the nearest hospital was in Sioux City, twenty-two miles away, patients had to go there when surgery was needed; then, weakened by the hospital experience, they would come by train to Sloan, probably facing a long ride in a lumber wagon over rough roads, to a home where good care was difficult or impossible. Father hoped now to be able to provide post-operative care for such patients in our home, and possibly to accommodate some minor surgical and non-surgical cases.

The trouble brought on the household by his first in-patient would have discouraged a less dedicated soul. The fall after we moved in, he was called to the hotel to see a transient who had all the symptoms of the grippe, which was prevalent at the time. The man had come from a cornhusking job over in Nebraska and hoped to find work near Sloan. Accommodations at the hotel were none too good even for a well person, and when the man became ill, the hotelkeeper begged Father to take him off his hands. Father talked it over with Mother, then brought him home and put him in a spare room.

That was on a Thursday night. Father looked in on the man the next morning, then was out on calls all day. At noon Mother took up a tray and a wash basin. When he had finished with his towel, she folded it and hung it up, then carried the basin out and left him with his lunch.

When Father came home toward evening he went directly to the man's room. He started to take his pulse—then stopped. There were a few red spots on the man's wrist, and, holding the lamp close to the patient's face, he found others. Cautiously he touched them; they felt like shot under the skin. For a moment he leaned back and studied the man, then asked as casually as he could, "Have you by any chance been exposed to smallpox?"

"Yes, I have," the man moaned. "I didn't know I had been exposed, I swear I didn't, Doc, but there was some smallpox around Decatur." He threw back the bed covers and tried to get up, but Father pushed him back, saying, "You've got to keep quiet; you have a high fever."

He still tried to get up. "I've got to get out of here or you will be quarantined. You can take me to Hornick for that night train and no one will know the difference. Where are my clothes?"

Father finally managed to quiet him, then said, "We will be quarantined, of course, if you have smallpox, and I'm pretty sure that is your trouble. I would have suspected it at first if I had known there was any around, but I think it has been fifteen years since I have known of a case in these parts, and your aching muscles and high temperature suggested the form the epidemic of the grippe is taking. Now here is the situation," he continued. "I have been thoroughly exposed and probably will contract the disease, so even if you left now I would be quarantined eventually in spite of anything we could do. But if you were to get on a train in your condition, you would expose others and probably start an epidemic. And if I knowingly let you do it, I would be in trouble with the law—real trouble."

Finally convinced, the man consented to stay. After talking with Mother, Father went directly to Dr. Hilts, who was town health officer. Then he telephoned the county health officer, who came down the next day. He confirmed the diagnosis and also helped make plans for those who might be in danger of contracting the disease. Being convinced that we children had not been exposed, he approved of our being taken away from home before the quarantine was put into effect.

It happened that Alice Lee, Edna's inseparable chum, had stayed all night with Edna Thursday night and Edna had gone home with her Friday night, so if one had been exposed so had the other. When they came home Saturday morning and were told of the trouble, Alice said, "Oh, goody! You can stay at our house until it's all over!" With the consent of her parents, it was so arranged.

Father had gone to call on an elderly neighbor, Mrs. King, after seeing the sick man settled on Thursday night, so now it became necessary to warn her. Learning that we children were not to be quarantined, she graciously offered to have me stay with her.

As for Charley, a neighbor boy had been in and out of our house all day with him. Dr. Hilts warned his parents and also arranged for them to keep Charley. Although Mother's sister, Mary Farley, lived nearby, and her son, Rolla, was just Charley's age, her husband's very elderly parents lived with them, and it seemed too much to add another small boy to their crowded household, especially one who had been in the house with a smallpox case.

Meanwhile, all who might have been involved were vaccinated. A spot on the arm was cleaned with alcohol, scratched until it bled, the serum applied, then rubbed in with what looked like a pen-shaped piece of bone. We children had been vaccinated before, but Mother, laughing off any possibility of her ever being exposed, had refused to have it done. Now she submitted readily and her reaction was unusually severe. As it turned out, the vaccination probably saved her life. It was said to prevent—and apparently did in her case—a "secondary fever" that usually proved more serious than the first stage of the disease.

The county health doctor, having done everything possible for our comfort and for the protection of the public, took the train for Sioux City, his last act being to tack a large, orange-colored sign on the house. Until then, the three doctors had worked quietly, but now the secret was out. There was smallpox in town! Pandemonium broke loose!

A few people hurriedly left town. Many stopped their work to huddle on street corners, often where they could watch our house. Some who had occasion to go down our street hurried by on the other side, with handkerchiefs held to their noses. Many and various charms were suggested as preventatives. The drugstore nearly sold out of asafetida, for many people had faith in a small piece of the ill-smelling gum tied in a little sack and hung on a string around the neck. Others hoped to avoid the disease by following fantastic diets.

A man who roomed over a store nearby wearied of keeping watch on our house by himself and went out to tell all who would listen, and there were a few, that Dr. Frear should be tarred and feathered! (For blocking a smallpox epidemic?) A neighbor on the other side of the street posted herself or a member of her family at her window day and night. Father could see her curtain flutter if he so much as went to the well; and always if he got up in the night he could see someone in the window, outlined against the lamplight.

Because we had left home so hurriedly, there was much to talk over, and as yet we had no local telephones to assist in communication. But Father—and for the first few days, Mother—watched for us children to pass the house, or we would call to them and could visit for a few minutes from the sidewalk while they stayed near the house, some thirty feet away. Needing warm underwear and nightclothes for the cold November weather, they asked us to purchase some for them. When we took the clothing to them, Father came out, and after a short visit we tossed the package into the yard and left. In minutes the report was over town that we were carrying things to and also away from the house.

Dr. Hilts usually talked to the folks as we did—from the sidewalk—but he also kept them supplied with medicines and food. After a few days he reported to Father that men in town had located a spot on the edge of town far removed from any residence and had hurriedly built a rough pest-house for the sick man; but he couldn't be moved until someone was found to care for him. Father knew a man out in the country who had had smallpox and Dr. Hilts asked him to go out and see if the man would come.

Father made the trip to get the nurse late at night to avoid meeting anyone, but the report went out that Dr. Frear was sneaking out at night and making calls as usual.

We children stayed away from school for two weeks, the period of incubation. By that time, the panic had subsided and we were accepted once more. Edna was having a real holiday with Alice. The Kings had been good to me, but they were elderly and their house was crowded, so when the Dan Utter family asked me to come there to stay and help with their three small children, I made the change.

At first, even during the worst of her illness from the vaccination, Mother had come to the window to wave when we were outside. About two weeks after the quarantine began, I stopped as I passed the house to watch Father hang out clothes. He did not use clothespins to fasten them to the line but tied towels by the corners, shirts by the sleeves. Mother did not come to the window and when I insisted on knowing why, Father finally admitted she was ill but said it might not be smallpox.

Then came the day when we called and watched the window in vain, for not even Father's face appeared. We hurried to Dr. Hilts and he confirmed our fears: both parents had smallpox! How desperately ill they were, especially Mother, we did not learn until much later. For several days she was delirious much of the time; sometimes when fully conscious she could hear incoherent ramblings from Father's bed. Too weak even to raise her head from the pillow, she was forced to listen without being able to console him or help in any way.

They were alone all this time—no nurse could be found for them—but during the most critical time a friend of Father's came to see them. A year earlier a Mapleton physician, Dr. J. H. Talboy, like Father, had contracted smallpox from an isolated case. Now he came by train, about sixty miles, and was able to give them not only advice and help but, even more, the hope and encouragement they so badly needed. He spent a day with them, leaving only when confident the crisis had passed.

One evening shortly after his visit, Mother was aroused from a nap. She thought she heard Charley call to her, but decided she had been dreaming or, possibly, was delirious. As she listened, however, she definitely heard sobbing outside the window, and a pathetic voice cried, "Mamma! Please, Mamma! Let me in!" Here was Charley's peaked little face pressed against the window-pane. He wanted to come home. He wanted to have smallpox with her. He wanted to die with her, rather than to stay away another night.

It was a difficult decision for Mother to make, with Charley at the window begging to come in, and even harder to explain to the boy. She wondered if it really were the right thing to do as, with a sinking heart, she persuaded the little fellow to go back and try it just a day or so longer. The next morning when Dr. Hilts stopped by, he was told of the incident, and he arranged for Charley to stay with Aunt Mary. The boy was contented with her and cousin Rolla.

The good people with whom he had been staying had a strong sense of duty, but some of their convictions seemed ill advised. Not for one moment was the little ten-year-old boy permitted to forget the threat that hung over him and, through him, over them as well. He was not allowed to play with, nor to sleep near, their son. He was constantly warned against exercise; his diet was restricted, supposedly to lessen the danger of contracting the disease, so that he had become thin and hungry as well as unhappy. Though Charley never complained of his treatment, after he came home, as he talked of things that had happened, Mother could see what the situation had been. Realizing how it must have worried them, she wondered that they had let him stay at all.

Mother's condition had begun to improve before they were able to get any help. Then on a Saturday morning the doorbell rang insistently. Father hurried to the window to warn any visitors away, but before he could say a word a small, sprightly woman called out, "You just unlock that door, Dr. Frear. I've had smallpox and I've come to help you folks out." Almost afraid to believe his good fortune, he admitted her. Without wasting a minute she came in, hung up her coat in the closet, and removed her white "fascinator" that covered her wispy gray hair, talking all the while. "We came in to do some trading this morning—first time in a month—and I heard how you folks didn't have a nurse, so I went to the store and got me a wrapper and a nightgown, and I says to the boys, 'You go on home and make out the best you can. I'm going to stay and take care of the Frears,' and here I am."

It wasn't their first meeting. She was one of those kindly souls who was always ready to go in and help where there was illness or trouble. Father sometimes found her there ahead of him when he arrived at a patient's bedside. She usually brought a kettle of soup or homemade bread and with them her own stock of ideas and remedies to use for the sick one. These usually included some of the favorite home remedies of the day: treacle and brimstone for a tonic; raw potato for burns; raw beef for a black eye; fat pork for the foot that had stepped on a nail. A chest cold was treated with a hot onion poultice; gangrene called for a dead chicken poultice, but one made with fresh cow manure was necessary for severe abdominal pains. A small but aggravating speck in the eye could be removed by the moist tip of a tongue.

Because of her well-meant interference, she and Father had clashed more than once, but all that was forgotten now. He almost embraced her, and had she suggested it right then, he doubtless would have submitted to one of her favorite "cures"—a dead chicken poultice for his smallpox pustules.

Now Mother could have the care she needed and he could get some much needed rest. During the past weeks, so many things had needed to be done that Father had disregarded his own condition in order to care for Mother and to keep things going; but now that they both could relax, the improvement that had already begun continued without interruption. Soon they were on the road to recovery.

Among the tasks that had been most demanding was the milking, for he couldn't let the cow suffer. Naturally, two people couldn't use all the milk, and of course they couldn't sell or even give it away. One method he found for disposing of it provided him with a little fun. There were five kittens in the barn at the time and Father trained them to sit in a row while he shot a stream of milk into each open red mouth in turn. He was quite proud of his accomplishment.

The mother, a large cat with white breast and feet and whorls of yellow on her back, had moved with us from the old house. She had been content until it was time for her kittens to be born, when she returned to deposit the litter in her favorite "nursery" under the old house. Later she carried each one to our barn by the nape of the neck and had just weaned them when our trouble began. On the day we were quarantined the old cat disappeared, and neighbors told us later that they had seen her on the sidewalk watching as the sign was nailed up. Father asked us girls to check on her, and we learned that she was back at the old house. The Joe Sloan family, who had moved there, said they would keep her. Not once did she come home until the Friday before Christmas.

117

That was the big reunion day for our family. The house had been thoroughly cleaned and fumigated, and many things were burned, including Father's large collection of medical journals and many of our old toys. My dolls were among the casualties.

The quarantine had been lifted on Wednesday but, knowing that our schoolmates might be afraid of us at first, we waited until Friday, when the two weeks' Christmas vacation began, to go home. We ran home from school that day, then ran from one dear, familiar place to another—our rooms, the barn, the office— all talking at once, until Mother called us to supper.

We bowed our heads while Father spoke the words that were so familiar, but his voice gave them a new meaning: "We thank Thee for all our many blessings." After he had finished we were very quiet.

Charley broke the silence: "Now if we only had the old cat we would be perfectly happy." Just then there was scratching and a loud "Me-eouw" at the back door. The old cat had come back, apparently as happy as we were that we were all together again.

Then in the spring misfortune sought us out again. The first day of Easter vacation an unseasonably cold spell had driven us children to huddle around the kitchen stove. Charley had been running a fever, and about noon we noticed that his face was brightly flushed. We ran to the office for Father, who at once diagnosed the trouble as scarlet fever. We knew that the children in a family who lived on the edge of town had the disease. Being both ignorant and stubborn, they had disregarded the quarantine, and the mother, dirty and germ laden, had gone about town as she pleased. Now Charley remembered that he had collided with her one day as she came through the post office door.

Mother and Charley were now isolated upstairs and Father moved into the office. He directed us girls in disinfecting the kitchen and gave us something to gargle. We followed his directions carefully except that we failed to dilute the medicine, a teaspoonful to a glass of water. We used it full strength and nearly choked, but it apparently killed any germs we might have had, for we didn't contract the disease. We girls cooked and carried food to the rest of the family during our period of incubation. Then Edna went to stay with Aunt Mary and I moved into the office with Father, while Mother and Charley took over the house.

Although he was not caring for a case of scarlet fever at the time, people assumed that Father had brought it home to Charley so, for a time, his practice fell off. This was fortunate in a way, for during that period he had a run of twenty-four boils on his right arm and was helpless for days. I cared for them under his direction as best I could, fed him, and helped him to dress and undress, all the while very conscious of the pain he suffered.

While his condition was at its worst, a stocky, thick-necked character we knew as "Slug" Smith came to get the doctor for his wife. Father was resting and I told the man that the doctor was not making any calls because he was sick.

"Whassa matter with him?" he demanded.

"He's got twenty-four boils on his arm—" I began.

"Ain't no blasted boils gonna let 'im off. You tell him to come see my wife right off," he blustered.

Just then Father came out to see who was there. Now Slug Smith was known to use patent medicines or go to quack doctors as long as he had any money, then call on Dr. Hilts or Father, either of whom would give him credit, though they knew they would probably never be paid; had it been possible, Father would probably have gone for the sake of the sick woman. He explained his difficulty, patiently, until the man shook his fist in Father's face and shouted, "You'll go to see my wife or I'll have you arrested!" Then Father really lost his temper and I listened astounded while he told his caller things about the law and doctors and certain patients, Slug Smith in particular, until the man backed toward the door and made a frightened escape.

Now, to return to the old cat; it would seem too much to expect even a doctor's pet to understand about quarantine, and of course she couldn't read signs. Nevertheless, we saw her sit on the sidewalk and watch while the yellow scarlet fever sign was being tacked to the house, then we saw her turn and walk away, just as the neighbors had seen her do when the smallpox sign went up. We learned that she had gone back to Joe Sloan's, and we never saw her again until the day the sign came down, when she came home again to stay. We had explained her absence during the smallpox siege by the fact that we children were away, but we were home during the scarlet fever quarantine, so we had no explanation to offer. Editor Frisbie heard of the incident and came to interview the feline prodigy, but she offered no comment. However, he checked with us and with the neighbors, and Tabby had quite a write-up in the *Sloan Star*.

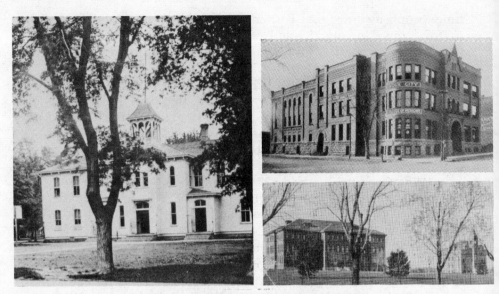

Frears studied and taught at the school in Sloan (left), Sioux City College of Medicine (above), and Morningside College.

Chapter 13

SCHOOL DAYS

THE END of the century brought other changes to our family besides the move to the new house. I entered high school in September, 1899; Edna was in her second year. Charley, recovering from scarlet fever, had been kept out of school so that he might build up a resistance to his earlier nervous trouble, but he went back to school in the fall of 1900, a normally active and healthy boy. He needed less care now, and we girls were quite able to take care of ourselves, so that Mother had some time to devote to church work. Beyond that, she cared little for social life; her main interests were her family and Father's practice.

And in the fall of 1900, even Father had a taste of school. He was devoting more time and thought than formerly to his practice in dermatology. Now he took a few weeks off and went to

120

Chicago to study X-ray diagnosis and treatment under the young Wagner brothers, who had developed a new type of X-ray machine. They even made one model with a handle that could be turned to generate a current for use where, as in Sloan, electricity was not available.

Father bought one of the machines and had it installed in the office. It was a vast improvement over the electric battery of ten years earlier, and it gave us children even a greater thrill to show it to our friends. For one thing, by turning it real fast we could flash colored lights or make a big spark jump six or eight inches from one shiny ball to another, all of which was impressive, though of no use to the doctor.

It is said that the Drs. Mayo of Rochester, Minnesota, bought one of the machines. Disgusted with such features as they considered merely "theatrical hooey," they called in an electrician to replace inessential parts with wooden plugs. Apparently they were more interested in its use for diagnosis, while Father used the rays mostly in treatment of skin diseases.

During his trip to Chicago, Father met Dr. Will Mayo, the older of the two brothers who had already become famous surgeons. He was impressed by the fact that they had their start as the sons of a doctor, and he came home with more enthusiasm than ever about the father-son relation in the medical profession. Charley listened, but the idea was too familiar to interest him, and he was too young to understand fully. I believe Father really tried not to put pressure on the boy to study medicine, but it was hard for him to refrain.

Possibly Father and Mother too, while they planned and sacrificed to give us an education, erred in that their ambitions for us followed too closely what they had wanted for themselves, but at least they gave us something to aim for: ideals, goals to reach. We were given every opportunity to study and encouraged to do our best; still we were never shamed or punished for doing less; we were never driven; and except on rare occasions, early bedtime took priority over studies.

In the same class with Edna and Alice, from their earliest school days, were several mischievous youngsters who, like the two girls, were never mean, and seldom deliberately disobedient, but who could think of ever so many things not covered by rules that would be fun to do. For example, there was no rule against bringing a pocketful of newborn pink mice to school, and letting them run about on the top of the desk. It was Earl Brader who carried that out, knowing that Miss Meyerhoff, the teacher, was so afraid of mice that she would not dare interfere. When he tired of playing with them, he simply bit off their heads and tossed them out of the window.

The girls had never been forbidden to shut Alice's big New-foundland dog in the recitation room during the noon hour. Ponto was harmless—toothless and friendly—but the five girls who came in, in single file after the noon session was called had no way of knowing that, and each one screamed as she stepped through the door and saw the huge black animal. The principal, who followed them, didn't scream; he turned pale and hurried his class back to assembly and out of danger.

Such pranks did not endear the children to their teachers, who were changed often in the lower grades, each one relieved when this group was promoted. But in high school, pupils met in the same assembly room for the entire four years. The staff looked about for ways to break up the crowd.

All were bright, some exceptionally so, had they cared to study. Alice had fair grades. Edna was working hard with her music. Mother's discipline had paid well: Edna had a good foundation and now, with a deep love for the piano and exceptional talent in performance, she could really make progress. She was generous in helping with church and school music. Unknown to her, when she practiced on a summer evening, our front lawn would be dotted with young folks sitting quietly while they listened. She had a small class of piano pupils, and even a waiting list, when she was fourteen, and was patient and thorough in her teaching.

There was nothing frivolous about Edna's attitude toward music, and, though she was always witty and fun loving, her behavior in general presented no serious problems for our parents. However, she refused to take her schoolwork seriously, so that her grades were only marginal. If she were kept back, she and Alice would be separated; also, Edna and I would be in the same class (I had skipped the second grade) and she might work to keep ahead of me. Thus reasoned the staff.

So at the end of their first year of high school, Alice was promoted and Edna was held back. The teachers may have had better control of the situation, but they still had problems. The girls found many ways to circumvent such minor handicaps as being seated a few rows apart, and Edna cared not at all if my grades were higher than hers, except that occasionally she concentrated on some subject just to show that she could beat me if she tried, and it wasn't necessary for her to try very hard.

Then, envious of the fun they were having, I tried a few tricks of my own, but I was not as clever as the older girls and always got caught; I found it easier to conform, as a rule, to the established pattern.

In 1903 Edna and I were graduated from high school. She knew exactly what she wanted to do—continue her study of music —but I had no definite plan. Secretly, I would have liked to become a writer, but I had no reason to think that I could make a career of writing. Sometimes I slipped away and started a story, but, afraid someone would find it and laugh at me, I always destroyed my efforts, and no one ever learned of my ambition.

Elocution appealed to me; I always liked to speak pieces, and my voice carried well; I had plenty of confidence; that fluttering in my stomach wasn't fear—it was excitement, and I loved it. But Father convinced me that there was no place for an elocutionist unless one went on the stage, and that would be unthinkable for one with my Methodist background who had been taught that even to attend the theatre was a sin.

A girl of sixteen really had little choice at that time, but Father told both Edna and me that, regardless of what vocation a girl followed, a college education should come first. He had already chosen the school for us. Morningside College in Sioux City was close by, comparatively inexpensive, and had a wholesome religious atmosphere, all of which appealed to him.

So I let my skirts down to the tops of my high-laced shoes, while Edna, since she was nearly nineteen, dropped hers to her insteps. The Gibson girl of the nineties still dictated the silhouette. A pompadour was called for; Edna's was a natural, and with the aid of a "rat" I managed to build one that was acceptable; I rolled up my stubby braid and tied it with a wide ribbon bow.

Carefully fitted pads had replaced the bustles of a few years earlier; falsies were ruffles and more ruffles on a pinnable piece of muslin. We made a number of each to round out the curves underneath the shirtwaists and skirts we had been sewing on all summer. We had blouses of cotton print for school, and colored silk or dainty white ones to be worn with sleek-fitted black skirts for best; and we had our white graduation dresses for parties. We were ready for college!

Father went with us to register. If he strutted a bit, surely he could be excused—the event really meant more to him than it did to us. And he was so happy to do this for us, so sure his plan was best, that Edna reluctantly gave up her hopes for a full-time music course and signed up for liberal arts. Under his watchful eye I signed up for all the science a freshman was allowed to take. Later Edna arranged for one piano lesson a week under a private teacher.

Mother had found rooms for us where we could do our own cooking and keep expenses down. Still the country doctor's daughters, we were kept supplied with produce brought in on account—maybe a slab of bacon or corned beef, a stewing hen, or a special treat of apples; we always had plenty of butter and eggs.

We saw Father often because of his connection with the Sioux City College of Medicine, where for a time he was secretary-treasurer, and for fifteen years he taught hygiene and dermatology. He came up every Thursday to meet his classes and usually was able sometime during the day to come out to Morningside to see us.

One Thursday not long after school started, he had something very special to discuss with me. Encouraged by my interest in helping him in the office, he had sometimes asked if I would like to come in the office with him, even suggesting that we might go to Chicago together and study, my work to be in bacteriology. I had had a vague picture of myself as office boy, janitor, bookkeeper, and possibly bacteriologist, whatever that was.

But this day he talked more about a comparatively new field for girls—doctor's assistant. If a girl understood the making of slides for the microscopic study of bacteria, and other laboratory techniques such as urinalysis, she could always get a good position. He'd had this in mind when he planned for me to specialize in science.

Then, too, he said there was the added possibility of work in a packing plant, or even for the government. The latter seemed a long way from home; I passed the packing plant going downtown from the college, always with a handkerchief held over my nose, so employment there made no appeal. But I listened as he went on to say I would need more histology than I could get at Morningside.

He told me about the class in histology that met on Thursday morning at the medical school, when I had only one class, college algebra, and on Monday, when I had none. He had already talked to the mathematics teacher, Professor Van Horne, who had told him that I could be excused that one day since I probably wouldn't pass anyway—a freshman seldom did—and the course would be repeated in the winter term. Medical school sounded rather exciting, so I agreed to take the course and went with him to register.

It might have been more exciting had I been a regular student or had my father not been on the faculty. In the early years it was the honest conviction of male medical students everywhere that women had no place in their school. They had various ways of smoking the girls out, and blowing cigar smoke in their faces was not the most objectionable. They could gang up to monopolize scarce materials, equipment, or working space; they could forget to pass along word about a change in schedule or a special assignment; and there were endless possibilities that ranged from embarrassing class discussions to nauseating clinics.

Possibly this school was broader than most medical colleges of the day. An advertisement of 1903 stated: "Women admitted on same conditions as men," and records show that two women had graduated in 1893, one the wife of Dr. H. A. Wheeler, a member of the faculty; and most of the succeeding classes had from one to three women.

I surely had no cause to complain about the boys. Maybe they just chose to ignore a girl in short dress and hair ribbon who blinked at them through thick lenses and didn't even understand their risqué jokes. Possibly they considered Father's position on the staff. But no doubt they were just the fine bunch of boys Father always thought them to be.

For the most part they were serious about medicine and, although the school was short on funds and furnishings, and enrollment was small, there was an opportunity for each one to work with an established physician and get experience and training that was possible for only a small percentage of students in the large universities.

The school was housed in the Y.M.C.A. building with its wide hallways and heavy staircases; the large, high-ceilinged rooms had the ornate paper on walls and ceilings, and the gas jets and heavily oiled floors characteristic of the period. The histology laboratory was fitted with handyman board tables and odds and ends of chairs, but there was a fair supply of microscopes and such other necessary equipment as was available at the time.

Five or six women worked at various times in the histology laboratory. There were the twins, plump, jolly, with a twist of auburn hair perched loosely somewhere near the crown of each head. You'd see one of them, sometimes both, at any class or discussion that was vital or interesting, taking copious notes. Father told me he couldn't tell them apart. When pressed further, he laughed and admitted that he hardly dared mark either one absent from class for fear she was the one who was present, and sometimes he was puzzled as to which one, if either, deserved a grade. One of the boys summed it up this way: "With all the notes they take to thrash over, what one doesn't know, the other will. Anyway, they'll want to practice together, so one diploma should do for both of them."

There was one tall, slender girl nearer my age, who had lovely long curls. She was quiet and dignified, ignored the boys, and took her work seriously. And there were one or two older women who probably were taking a refresher course—they did not come to the laboratory regularly.

My favorite of the girls was Martha McCullough. As near as I could determine, Martha was studying medicine to be near her adored brother, Tom, who was a senior. I loved her lilting Irish brogue and her warm Irish heart. She seemed to sense my shyness and took me under her wing, and through her I gained some sense of belonging.

One day I went with Father to visit his hygiene class. When we entered the door at the back of the sparsely-furnished classroom most of the students had assembled and were seated, watching a performance by one of the boys who was better known as a clown than as a top student. With his hands clasped behind him, his head down and eyes always on the floor, he walked across the front of the room with short, quick steps, then turned. Back and forth he went as he talked: "To see a woman fifty pounds overweight mincing along in shoes three sizes too small is not only disgusting, it is pathetic." It was a favorite theme of Father's but one need not know that to realize whom the boy impersonated. I looked at Father to see how he took it. His sides shook with suppressed laughter. Some of the students saw him and were almost hysterical as the young man continued. "She is ruining her posture and laying herself open to many serious internal diseases. To get properly-fitted shoes one should stand with all the weight on one foot and trace the outline, then insist on getting shoes that conform to this measure."

Just then the student looked up and saw us in the doorway. Embarrassed almost to tears, he slid into a seat in the back of the room, and amid a round of applause Father took his place and began to speak. "It is gratifying to know that a student has paid close attention to the subject matter as well as to the instructor." This was greeted with laughter, and as he proceeded with the lecture, his little mannerisms brought a smile now and then, but he had the respectful attention of the class.

Now in presenting a subject as sweeping in scope as hygiene, one could include many things, and Father gave a share of his attention to the use of tobacco and alcohol, also to a pet peeve of his and a common nuisance with which a doctor has to contend— patent medicines. Although it may have been a bit off the course, he could not resist telling the class of a personal experience with the latter, since it also tied in with the use of alcohol.

While Father did prescribe medicines containing alcohol, especially where it was used as a necessary solvent, he advocated the practice of total abstinence and aligned himself with others who worked for the same principles. However, one group of people, a sect that had separated from the church because they said it was too worldly, failed to get his cooperation. He objected to their fanatical views on many religious questions, and their noisy demonstrations in meetings offended his conservative Presbyterian sensibilities; on the problem of drinking he had reason to doubt the sincerity of some of their leaders.

"A personal element entered into our relations too, one which you may be called upon to face," he told his class, "for we did not see alike on the practice of medicine. One of their number had a profitable sideline selling a patent medicine—we'll call it I-CUR-ALL—and for many of them the procedure had become to 'trust in the Lord and take a little I-CUR-ALL along with it.' and call the doctor only as a last resort. I repeatedly warned clients against the use of this nostrum, but some thought my objection was due solely to its having robbed me of some of my practice.

"On one occasion a well-meaning woman even offered my twelve-year-old daughter some I-CUR-ALL for her cold," he went on. "The child had sense enough to refuse, whereupon the woman said, 'Oh, I know your pa don't approve of it, but it's too bad, for you've got catarrh and I-CUR-ALL would cure it.' "

He went on to tell of a big temperance rally staged by these people who had hired a well-known temperance speaker for the affair. Father did not work with them nor did he attend. "But I wished afterward I had gone," he said. "Everyone was talking about it next day. It seems the lecturer told his audience that some of them might be imbibing without realizing it. To illustrate his point he took out a bottle of I-CUR-ALL and proceeded to analyze it, and showed them that the content was 20 percent alcohol. I doubt if the erstwhile dealer was surprised, but he was embarrassed, and as word of the demonstration spread around town, he was laughed right out of business. That was unfortunate for him too, because there was no saloon in Sloan, and once the alcoholic content became known, I-CUR-ALL was in great demand."

Although I visited Father's lectures and occasionally one of the other freshman classes, I avoided the advanced ones; but one time I made an exception and took in part of the class in anatomy. This was held in a large, well-lighted room with seating arranged so that a fairly large group could see the long table at the front of the room. They met just before our histology class, and sometimes I waited for Martha McCullough in the hall outside.

One morning as I stood there, Carl McCaig, a tall good-looking senior whom I knew slightly—and feared more, because of his biting sarcasm—came from the classroom before dismissal and saw me waiting. We spoke as he passed, then he turned and motioned to me. Speaking in a low voice he said, "Miss McCullough said if I saw you to tell you to come on in the classroom. Now don't knock—you'd disturb them. Wait a few minutes, 'til I get out of hearing, then go in as quietly as you can. Watch that door knob it squeaks." Carl went on down the hall with a twisted smile on his face, but I thought nothing of that, from Carl.

I determined to make no noise. Dr. Dales had that anatomy class and I didn't want to incur his displeasure. He had a long, slender face and a high forehead that ran pink and shiny clear to the back of his neck. He had large, dark eyes behind owlish lenses and a perpetual grin that could mean anything to one who didn't know him well.

Stealthily I turned the knob, taking my time. Then as I started slowly to open the door, a hinge squeaked, so I stepped inside quickly and closed it. Every eye in the room, including the professor's, turned on me. There was an awful silence for a moment, then everyone laughed, simply howled, except Dr. Dales, who grinned—horribly, I thought—at me. I looked from his face to the table in front of him. There lay a cadaver, brown and ghastly. The scalp had been cut back, and from appearances, they had been dissecting the brain. A row of boys stood close by in a semicircle; other students, including the girls, stood behind them on chairs.

So Carl McCaig thought he'd play a joke on me and scare the wits out of me, did he? Well, I'd show them that a doctor's daughter could take it. I walked past the body on the table with a boldness I didn't quite feel. A titter went around the room as I climbed up on a chair beside Martha. She put a protective arm around me and the class turned its attention to the anatomy lecture.

When I saw Father again he said, "I hear you visited Dr. Dales' anatomy class."

"Yes," I said, and laughed. "Carl McCaig thought he'd give me a big scare but it didn't work."

He chuckled. "The joke wasn't on you at all," he said; then he explained. It seems that the body Dr. Dales had been working on had not been held for the length of time specified by law. Some of the boys, chiefly Carl, had hinted that the authorities were aware of it but, knowing their tendency to joke, Dr. Dales had made light of it. I had played right into their hands. Carl's instructions and timing had been perfect, and when I slipped so quietly into the room, both Dr. Dales and the class had thought it was the law. He told Father that he had had the worst scare of his life. He never forgot it, and Father said later that Dr. Dales retold the incident every time my name was mentioned. So at least my brief attendance at medical school had not gone unnoticed.

Back at Morningside, Edna's talent and her love for music were becoming recognized, but her interest in her studies did not improve. Probably her neglect of her assignments was deliberate; the only way she could contrive to get permission for a full-time music course was to drop out or flunk some studies so that there would be fewer classes available for her. Later, even Father admitted that Edna knew what was best for her and, secretly proud of her independence, he consented to her devoting all her time to music in the spring term.

We moved during our first winter to the home of Mrs. Ella Toenjes, who taught in the grade school, and here we shared expenses and housework with her family. Her two daughters, Ella and Carlotta, who were friends of ours and about our own age, studied violin and cello and, like Edna, took their work seriously. For two years Edna played accompaniments for them, and the three were in great demand for programs at the college; they also gave concerts in small nearby towns. Then the Toenjes family moved to Chicago. A year later Edna joined them there; she had been granted a scholarship at the Chicago Musical College.

Since I was alone, during the next two years I lived near the college. I continued with the science courses; Father still hoped I would become a doctor's assistant. Then on one of his visits to the college, in the biology laboratory where I spent most of my time, he became acquainted with Lon Hawkins, the six-foot-three, redheaded assistant.

He and Lon liked each other from the first meeting; in fact, I believe Father sensed a certain trend before I did, for he no longer talked about my career in science.

Lon graduated in 1906. He had accepted a fellowship at Ohio State University for the following year, but he spent the summer in Morningside, since he lived there with his parents. As he usually did during his vacations, he worked at inside finishing with a local builder—he had been obliged to make his own way throughout his college course.

I stayed for the six weeks summer school to make up some required nonscience credits, and assisted in the biology laboratory. Lon and I had had a few dates during the spring—not many, because he had a heavy schedule and little to spend on good times. But during the summer we were together often, usually rowing on the Big Sioux River after picnicking at Riverside Park.

The laboratory seemed pretty empty the next year. I had come to depend on Lon's help and advice more than I had realized. But I heard from him often and was proud when, before the end of the year at Ohio State, he was asked to come to Washington, D.C., at once, to work with the Department of Agriculture.

I was graduated in 1907, still undecided about my lifework. Dr. R. B. Wylie, who had been Lon's major professor and mine, was now at the University of Iowa and wanted me to take graduate work there, with the prospect of a scholarship, but I was tired of studying, and Father wanted me to stay home and rest and be both companion and helper to him and Mother. Then toward fall, Mr. Ralston came and asked me to teach their school over in the hills, and I decided to accept. Teacher training had not been included in my course, but my college degree entitled me to a temporary certificate, so I became a teacher, in name at least.

Meanwhile, Lon had found government work much to his liking; he wrote that living in Washington was pleasant and interesting, and he hoped that I would share it with him. When he came home for a visit in October we became engaged. At last I had decided on a career, one of which Father thoroughly approved.

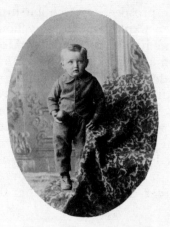

Son of a doctor and himself a doctor-to-be, Charley Frear, age one and a half, eyes the photographer's birdie anxiously.

Chapter 14

BABIES—TEN DOLLARS DELIVERED

OFTEN when Father had delivered a baby boy, the mother, in a burst of relief and gratitude, would ask, "Dr. Frear, what is your first name?"

He had an answer always ready: "Edwin. It's a fine old name. Three babies have already been named for me. Two of them died, and the other had fits." The mother would laugh, and choose another name.

It was not strange that they did not know his given name. He always signed himself simply "E. D. Frear," and few people in Iowa ever had known him as Ed. His friends, knowing how he disliked to be called "Doc," called him "Doctor," as Mother did.

Strangely enough, he was pleased when a baby was named "Frear"; I have even known him to suggest it. A few little girls were named for Edna, but none for me—he refused to admit Cora was my name.

Altogether in his twenty-six years of country practice, Father delivered about twelve hundred babies. The usual fee for pre-natal care and delivery was ten dollars when birth was normal and distance to the home not too great. Hospital confinements were of course unknown among rural women of the early day. Indeed, when he had started practice in Salix, most women had depended on midwives. As his practice grew, confinement cases had increased proportionately, and when he moved to Sloan, where there were already two doctors, women had grown used to special care and were quick to call on a doctor.

Among Father's deliveries were multiple births, of course, but they included only one set of triplets—two boys and a girl. Then, too, abnormal babies sometimes appeared. One little girl arrived with extra fingers and toes—twelve of each, the extra ones being abnormal and out of line. Father had snipped off the extra fingers and one of the toes, when the baby's grandmother saw what he was doing. Screaming, she snatched the baby from him and refused to allow him to remove the other toe. The child grew up with an extra toe; in order to be fitted with a shoe she had to learn to fold that one toe, just so, underneath the others.

Less fortunate was the infant born with stiff, straight arms, without elbow joints. Father wanted to cut wedges where the joints should have been, so her arms would be bent rather than straight. If done at the time, it would have been a comparatively simple operation. The young mother could see the advantage; it would have brought the child's hands up so she could reach her face; it would have enabled her to feed herself, comb her hair, hold a book in front of her eyes to read, and do many other things impossible with hands always held at arms' length. Again it was the grandmother who interfered, and the young mother, too weak to oppose her and insist on the operation, was obliged to let the opportunity pass.

This family lived some distance from Sloan, and possibly the argument about the arms made them reluctant to call Father again, so he did not keep in touch with them and had almost for-gotten the case. Then about twelve years later he was called to the home again. While he was mixing medicine for his patient, he saw a barefoot girl who sat on the floor, her arms held straight out in front of her while she tried to draw a picture. His attention was first attracted to her when a persistent fly kept alighting on her head and she brushed it off deftly, not with her hand but with her foot. As he watched her he recalled the baby born without elbow joints.

On the floor beside her was a plate with a cup of milk and some cookies. Wondering how she would handle them, he glanced at her from time to time. Presently he saw her pick up the cup with the toes of one foot, drink the milk and set the cup down, hardly lifting her eyes from her drawing. In the same way, she picked up a cooky and ate it. Apparently she was equal to any occasion for the present; possibly she had an advantage in being able to use both hands and feet simultaneously, but he wondered how she managed in the winter, when shoes and stockings were a necessity.

Fortunately, such children were a rare exception; most of the infants he delivered were normal and husky like their outdoor-living, corn-fed parents, and they were a joy as well as a challenge to Father. He and I shared our love for the tiny newcomers, and while it was out of the question to take me with him on confinement cases, whenever possible he took me later to see the new babies. I adored them, even though, looking at their red faces and egg-shaped heads, whether bald or covered with a thatch of long dark hair, I sometimes wondered why their mothers were so proud of them. But usually I was speechless with awe, so I seldom said anything that might hurt the mother's feelings.

As I look back, it seems to me Father must have considered this as part of the preparation for the life of a woman, and he did not spare me the less happy side of the picture. I remember that he took me to see the Chesley twins when they were only a few hours old. They were the seventh and eighth children of a shiftless father and a beaten, dragged-out mother, and there had been little preparation for their coming. They made a pathetic picture, the mother lying on a sagging bed which had neither sheets nor pillowcases, the babies on a soiled blanket spread across the foot of the bed. The scrawny little girl was pinned into a dress belonging to a four-year-old sister; the even thinner boy was wrapped in an older brother's blouse. They had no shirts, and only rags torn to size for diapers. The townspeople had grown weary of doing things for this family, but Mother felt the situation was an emergency, so she called on some of the neighbors for help and managed to find a few shirts and dresses, and some flour sacks for diapers; she took them to the family, with sheets from her own shelves. Fortunately, it was summer and warmer clothing was not so badly needed.

It is doubtful if Mrs. Chesley enjoyed a ten-day lying-in period, at that time considered the minimum for proper adjustment and recovery from the ordeal of childbirth. Of course two weeks rest was even better, with six weeks of being careful; grandmothers who never heard the term "baby-sitting" took on the cooking and all the care of the family as well as of the baby. The latter included such things as boiling every diaper each time it was used. If Grandma was not available, a strong country girl could usually be hired for two dollars a week, with no provision for overtime or coffee breaks.

It is possible that all this precaution was necessary following a pregnancy in the nineties. The expectant mother was told by her family and friends, if not by her doctor, "Now remember you must eat for two!" and she was warned against exercise. Even walking was considered too strenuous by some; besides it was indiscreet to be seen on the street after her condition began to "show." To further encourage inactivity, she must sit around and sew on the layette that the well-dressed baby of the time must have, since there were few ready-made baby clothes available.

Dresses for "best" were at least a yard long, and the lower part was encircled with rows of tucks and inserted lace, possibly hemstitched, worn over a long slip, also lace trimmed. A woman might use the sewing machine, if one was available, rather than doing all this by hand, but she would be criticized by her fastidious friends; she took a risk, too, pedalling a sewing machine in her condition.

There were simpler dresses for everyday, but the baby—girl or boy—must be dressed completely every day. Never could it lie with only shirt and diaper, even in the hottest weather. That simply was not done! And when the dresses and slips were ready, there were the nightgowns, the pinning blankets and receiving blankets and crib blankets, and crocheted or embroidered sacques and caps and bootees to be made.

And so, some fifteen pounds overweight, with muscles flabby and sluggish from lack of exercise, the young woman of the nineties was delivered of a baby larger by two pounds than its counterpart of the 1960s, and possibly a ten-day rest in bed was a blessing if not a necessity.

If added to the usual labor and childbirth were the excitement and worry that confronted Mrs. Alfred Taylor, a farmer's wife living east of Sloan, even more time might be required in order to restore frayed nerves. The Taylors had a small farm with the usual fields of corn and wheat, two cows, and a flock of chickens; but Mr. Taylor had also developed a small project raising bees and selling honey.

Their house was small and they already had four children, so he was adding a bedroom which he had hoped would be ready when the new baby arrived, but wet weather had hindered the work. They sent for Father, and as he drove into the lane, he could see the new addition. He observed that the roof was on, but the siding was on only as far as the rafters, which left an open space under the eaves, and neither windows nor doors were hung.

A boy ran out of the house to tie Father's team. Alf Taylor met him at the door with a worried look on his face, and on his head a straw hat draped with mosquito netting. He led Father into the new room, where he found his patient in bed wearing a sunbonnet and veil. Mr. Taylor pointed to the ceiling, but Father's attention had already been drawn there by a buzzing sound made by a dozen or more honeybees. "Gosh all fishhooks!" he exclaimed, then looked through the window opening where a swarm of bees attempted to cluster under the eaves, not twelve feet from the foot of the bed. Around and around, counterclockwise they circled. obeying their God-given instinct to join their queen and help build a new colony. They had a little trouble because the cluster hung so near the side of the house that some lost their way and flew inside.

Father turned to Mrs. Taylor. "Don't you want us to carry you into another room?"

"It's too late. We couldn't—" She stopped as a labor pain seized her.

Taylor said hopelessly, "They started coming just as the pains got bad and it was too late to move her. And there wasn't a thing I could do about it."

"We'll make out," Father said and hurried to the kitchen, where a neighbor woman waited on him while he disinfected his hands and slipped on a clean white coat. When he returned, the bees were coming by the dozens, but most of them found their way out again.

"Don't fight them and you're probably safe," the man said, "but Gawd help us if anything disturbs them."

Keeping his patient well covered, Father prepared her for delivery. Once a bee got too close and, without thinking, he brushed at it with his arm, so that he was stung on the head. He never looked up while Taylor pulled out the stinger and the neighbor applied damp soda, and when they put a netted straw hat on him, he accepted it without protest. The humming sound increased, but he ignored it.

Soon the veiled doctor delivered the veiled patient of a nine-pound baby. A veiled neighbor waited with more mosquito netting while he spanked the small red bottom. With her first lusty cry, the baby girl was hurried to the kitchen, where a clothes-basket was ready with warm bricks and still more mosquito netting.

It was all over in an hour. The last bee had joined the cluster and all was quiet except for a low, contented hum. The young mother wept with relief. Her husband patted her shoulder awkwardly. "You see if you can't get some sleep now, and later I'll carry you into the other room to stay while I take care of the bees," he promised. "I've got an extra hive in the barn."

They named the baby "Beatrice," but they called her just plain "Bee."

Such incidents were all in the day's work for the country doctor. But after Father moved to the city in 1908 he wanted to break away from the demands of general practice and, even more, of obstetrics, and devote himself to office work in the field of dermatology. However, he had brought with him the country doctor's sympathy and understanding of the whole pattern of family life, so that people came to him because they could talk freely with him.

Occasionally some woman overestimated the appeal of her problem and learned to her surprise that, though sympathetic, he did not always see things her way. There was the case of Mrs. Williams, who had lived near Sloan and had known the doctor all her life. She had married in her thirties, and both she and her husband had regretted that they had no children. When she was about forty she had not felt well for a few weeks, and in fun had told her husband that she thought she was pregnant. He was so thrilled and happy that she kept up the deception for a while. Then he had to go to California to attend his father's funeral and settle the estate; he expected to be gone about two months. When she decided not to accompany him he assumed it was because of her "condition," and she did not deny it, because she had a big idea. Confiding in Father, she asked him to find her a suitable new baby, and on Mr. Williams' return, to help her pass it off as their own child.

The lady reasoned that she could just pay Father two or three hundred dollars and all would work out fine. She made a big point of the pride and joy her husband would have in the child, and that seemed to her to excuse the deception, but Father did not agree. He told her that with her husband's consent he would try to find them a child for adoption, but under no circumstances would he deceive a man in such a matter.

In striking contrast, he had an occasional request for an abortion. One had its amusing side, though at the time he failed to see it. A Mrs. Hale, a former patient who had been just an average, hardworking housewife, had recently received an inheritance. Now she was trying to break into social circles that had previously been denied to her. One day she brought her daughter to see him.

The lovely Eva had married well. Father knew and admired the popular young Morningside couple. They entertained charmingly and also were in demand because of their musical talents. They had been an asset to the ambitious mother, who herself had little to offer, but who had been included in many of their social events. Father admired the progress Mrs. Hale had made; it had not been easy to acquire that slender figure, easy carriage, and modulated voice; and she was tastefully dressed.

But his admiration ceased when she stated her errand. Her little Eva was pregnant, she said, and as he knew, she was too frail and inexperienced to be burdened with the responsibility of a baby. They had come to him because they knew how kind he was, and that he would understand.

He understood, alright. She did not want to become a grandmother. It occurred to him that a baby's soft body really might be out of place on that smartly tailored shoulder, its little hands and mouth exploring that professional make-up and hairdo. Furthermore, all the gains she had made socially would be threatened if Eva withdrew, even temporarily, from her social activities, just as her mother was becoming recognized. But as he looked at the younger woman, watching him with appealing, tear-swollen eyes, he felt sure that she would be happy with the only answer he could give them.

He tried to reason with the woman. He told her that not

only was an abortion illegal, but that it would endanger the health and possibly even the life of her daughter. He politely but firmly told her that under no circumstances would he perform such an operation.

Now she tried being coy, and said sweetly, "Now, Dr. Frear, don't be difficult. You see, I've known you for years and you're always kind and helpful. Now I'm just asking a small favor." She paused and reached for her purse. "And I'm ready to pay you well, and in advance too. And I'm sure that you can use the money."

Bent over her checkbook, she did not see that he was shaking with anger. Eva, apparently frightened, was crying, but Mrs. Hale went on, "There! I've made this for five hundred dollars. If that isn't enough, I'll give you more." She laid the check on his desk. His answer was to take her by the arm, lift her from her chair, and practically shove her out the door.

Eva followed, pausing only long enough to give him a low-spoken but fervent thank-you. He tore the check to bits and tossed it in the wastebasket. And at the time he didn't know where his rent money was coming from, not to mention the expense of sending a boy to medical college.

As a rule, it was a woman who consulted Father about the problems of having, or not having, babies, but he had one case that was an exception. A young friend and former neighbor, Grant Billstead, used to drop in the office occasionally for a chat, and often spoke of their disappointment at not having a family. Apparently he wanted advice, but there was little Father could do for them, especially since his wife, Grace, had never consulted him as a physician. He did, however, suggest that Grant have his wife consult a certain gynecologist; he also offered to help them find a child for adoption.

He learned later that Grace flatly refused to consider either suggestion, insisting that she was all right and that she would have a baby of her own. Father understood that Grace's sister, Mrs. Hartler, had had her only child when she was nearly thirty. He had met the Hartlers on their visits to the Billsteads with their lovely daughter, Elinore, who often spent her vacations with her aunt and uncle.

When Grace passed her thirtieth birthday, she became moody and her husband was worried. Then he learned that she had made baby clothes and had shown them to her friends. When he asked her about it she became hysterical. Deeply concerned, he came to Father, who studied the problem from all angles, still handicapped by lack of cooperation from Grace.

At that time, Father had a case of a young stenographer who was about to have a baby, the child of her employer who was a lawyer with good professional standing and a lovely family. Both were eager to have the baby placed for adoption in a good home and left all details to Father. The mother preferred never to see the child.

When the baby arrived, Father immediately called the Billsteads. This was an emergency, he said—a lovely baby girl was refused by both parents. Would they consider caring for it until he could find a home for it? He was sure it would be only a few days. As he had expected, once they had taken the baby into their home, they would not consider giving her up. A chain of circumstances, including her having shown the baby clothes, made it possible for them to pass the child off as their own, even to the Hartlers, and Elinore was delighted with her little cousin, Gloria.

There followed two happy years for the Billsteads. Then came business losses; to regain them Grant overworked and succumbed to an attack of pneumonia. At the end of another year, Grace found herself with a tottering business, which she alone could not save, and the little girl to provide for. Rather than take outside work that would keep her away from Gloria, she took in laundry, rented out most of her house, and made many other sacrifices, all of which taxed her strength.

One time she brought the little girl in for Father to prescribe for a burn on her hand. Realizing what a struggle she was having, he cautioned her about her own health and offered to find a good home for the child. Tearfully, her lips trembling, she asked, "Dr. Frear, haven't I lost enough? Would you take my baby, too?"

After that she avoided him. When he saw her again it was at the request of neighbors who found her ill and sent for him, but it was too late for him to save her. From what neighbors told him, life for her had been even harder than he had realized, but he found that little Gloria, now five years old, was a happy, robust child, obviously well fed and cared for, while her mother had neglected her own health to give to the little girl.

The niece, Elinore, now married and living in the East, came with her husband to take charge. There was no hesitancy about the child; she would, of course, give her a home—she loved her as a sister.

Father had kept the secret of Gloria's background until now, but it did not seem right to let the young couple take the child under the impression that she was a cousin, so he told them her story. Elinore listened quietly, then she asked, "Would her real parents want her?"

"Definitely not. And neither one knows where she is. They left everything to me."

"And no one else has a claim to her?"

"Not a soul. But you are young, Elinore, and will have a nice family of your own."

"We hope so; still, Gloria belongs to me," Elinore said firmly. "As you say, there is no blood tie between us, but there is another tie that is very strong; for like Gloria I was a child of—of unfortunate circumstances."

"What do you mean? Surely you are not saying the Hartlers were not your real parents? Why, there is such a strong family resemblance. . . ."

She was watching him closely. "Dr. Frear, had it ever occurred to you that I resembled Aunt Grace more than I did Mom? Or that I was tall like Uncle Grant rather than short like my folks?"

Father stared at her, unbelieving. Was she telling him that the Billsteads were her real parents? She said quickly, "Please don't judge them too harshly. They were just kids, only sixteen. And at any time after they were married, they would have faced the world with the truth and claimed me as their own child, only they thought everyone would be hurt."

"How long have you known?" he asked.

"Oh, I began to notice resemblances and ask questions when I was ten or twelve, and when I was fifteen they told me the whole truth. Aunt Grace was wonderful. She talked frankly with me; she wanted to help me avoid trouble, and I could always confide in her. I could have gone to live with them then, but that would have left Mom and Dad alone. And we kept hoping Aunt Grace would have a baby—she never did give up."

"You're right about that," Father said, "and you have explained things that had puzzled me. Well, Gloria is a lovely child. healthy and well behaved. And I can assure you her background is of the best. Only you and I and your husband need ever know her story, or yours. May God bless all of you."

Father's interest in the problems of the Billsteads was, of course, outside the demands of the practice of medicine, but so were many other opportunities for service that he enjoyed. Often someone who was discouraged or worried came in on a pretext of wanting professional help, when his real need was for a sympathetic listener. His practice not being heavy, Father could usually devote time to consider all phases of a patient's needs, and charity patients were often sent to him by nuns and deaconesses.

One young woman had been referred to him by a deaconess, who surely had not been told the true nature of her problem. The girl was poorly dressed and timid, but at first she tried to put on a bold front. She said, as though it had been rehearsed, "I've heard that you are a very understanding person and I've come to you because I need help." Then she became embarrassed and Father had to coax her story from her. He could see that she had worked hard and worried more. He saw something else, too, but waited for her to tell him.

It seems that about five years before this she had run away from her home out in Nebraska to marry a man to whom her father and mother strongly objected. They had come to Sioux City to live, and she soon found out the man was even worse than her parents had feared. Six months before coming to see Father, she had divorced him, but he had been coming back to annoy her. It was evident that she was afraid of him, and now she was three months pregnant.

Her husband had never supported her. She had worked as a waitress days and had done office cleaning at night until her health had broken. Recently, another man had been taking her out and they were about to be married, when she had discovered that a baby was coming. She felt it was impossible for her to go on alone—she needed someone to make a home for her and to protect her from her former husband; but Father suspected from what she said that the second man was little better than the first. She had been honest enough to tell this man of her condition, and he refused to take care of another man's child. She said she had a hundred dollars saved up and she could pay; there just mustn't be any baby to interfere with her marriage.

This doctor who had practically thrown a wealthy woman from the office for a similar request sat back in his squeaky swivel chair and listened sympathetically to the girl before him. He could see that she was from a good home and he was thinking of that home as he encouraged her to talk. Finally he said in his kindly way, "I can see that you have had a hard time. I hope better days are ahead for you, and I would be glad to help you. But if I take your case there are certain conditions you will have to meet."

"I'll do anything you say, doctor—anything!" she said.

"Good!" he said. "Now you know of course that what you ask is illegal except in certain emergencies, so you must promise not to tell anyone that I will take your case or even that you have talked it over with me. We must have absolute secrecy. Do you agree to that?"

"Of course I do. I don't want it known either."

"All right. Now the first thing I want you to do is to write to your parents, this very night. You are to give them your correct address, for I understand they don't know where you are. Aside from that, write anything you please."

"Oh, no, Doctor, I can't do that! It has nothing to do with the case. And my folks don't want to hear from me." She started to cry. "After all these years, it's better to let them forget me. I'll do anything but that."

"My dear child, I am a parent," he said quietly. "I have two daughters. Both are married to good men and they are a great comfort to me, but I still would love them if they ignored me entirely. And if they left me as you have done I would pray every day for word from them, if only to know where they were."

He paused for a moment, since she seemed to be thinking over what he had said, then he went on: "Now of course I could be mistaken about your parents; however, if I am to take care of you, I should have your next of kin listed on my records. Since you are divorced from your husband, I must be able to get in touch with your parents. And in any case, you must write to them as my first condition." He stood up with a gesture of dismissal. "Do this tonight and call me or come in a week from today." Tearfully she half-promised, and left.

He was not surprised to hear from her a few days later that she was going home for a week but would see him on her return. Of course she did not come back. He had played a hunch and won. He had a letter from the girl, but it was her mother who wrote him later of the arrival of the fine baby boy, and who, about two years later, sent a picture of the little fellow, which Father had framed and hung above his desk. In the accompanying letter, the mother told of the girl's marriage to a fine young man who had been her high school sweetheart, and closed her letter with: "We still pray for you and thank God that our daughter took her troubles to a doctor who, like the Great Physician, heals a soul while he saves a life."

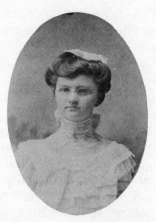

Suddenly, Cora was a grown-up young
lady. There is little evidence of her tomboy
days in her Class of '03 graduation photo.

Chapter 15

TRANSITION

D URING the year after I was graduated from college, I
taught rural schools—one over in the hills in the fall and
spring, and in the winter, a small school four miles
southwest of town so close that I could stay home and drive to
school each day, except in stormy weather. Edna was studying
music on a scholarship in Chicago, and Charley had started college
at Morningside. It was to be my last year before my marriage, and
I enjoyed the leisurely hours with Father and Mother.

It was a year of transition for all of us, for it was evident that
Father would soon have to give up country practice. Irregular
meals and sleep and one strenuous trip after another, often with
no rest between, had taken a toll of his health. He had spells of
indigestion, his blood pressure was high, and his hearing was failing due to exposure to cold and wind.

In January of 1907 he had started an office in Sioux City,
where he shared waiting room and facilities with a masseur, and
the results had encouraged him to think he could make a success of

city practice. A graduate from the medical school helped him at Sloan, making the long trips that were too tiring for Father.

He was concerned, too, about Mother—he wanted to make things easier for her. Many modern conveniences were not even available in Sloan. And while they both loved their rural patients and friends, he had made many friends in the city, and he knew Mother would make a place for herself in a new environment.

Then, too, he looked forward to a time when he would have more leisure: evenings at home with Mother, and time to read and to indulge his urge to write. He had always been interested in history, and in social problems, especially as they were related to the use of tobacco and alcohol, and he felt he might do something worthwhile by telling of his own observations and convictions. In this Mother encouraged him.

Another factor entered into the situation; about that time a movement was under way to standardize medical colleges, and when the Sioux City school found they could not meet the new requirements, they closed their doors. That eliminated the free clinics where students had brought in skin cases for study and treatment under Father's supervision. There was no other dermatologist in a large territory, and, unless Father became established soon, someone might take advantage of the opening, and he would find himself with a competitor.

The young doctor who had been helping him at Sloan had another place in mind, and now, as a definite step toward the change, Father looked about for a permanent assistant who would make the longer drives and be in charge of the office afternoons while Father was away, and who would be interested in taking over the entire practice, if and when Father decided to leave Sloan. Dr. Lee Prescott, who had been located for a short time in Hornick, was the answer to this problem. He was a friend of Dr. Lacy, which made the arrangement even more agreeable. Now Father rented better office rooms in the city and went up every day, train service making it possible to reach his office by noon and be back home by six o'clock in the evening.

The work grew steadily, though slowly, made up largely of cases referred to him by doctors who were formerly his students. However, one of the worst cases to come to his city office was sent by another member of the faculty, a well-known surgeon who, at the request of a friend, had accepted a case of what appeared to be a minor skin eruption.

When this doctor saw the patient for the second time, he was so alarmed at the progress the disease had made that he sent her to Father. By the time Father saw her, the girl's face was entirely covered by a mass of overlapping sores, which he diagnosed as tuberculosis of the skin.

The patient was blue-eyed, golden-haired Alma Johnson, a fifteen-year-old girl with a round face and a pleasant voice, although she was shy and had little to say. Her parents were of sturdy Swedish stock and lived about thirty-five miles from Sioux City. Her father worked for the railroad as a section boss, and a pass made possible Alma's trips to the city for her treatments.

It so happened that at the same time Father had two other patients with similar skin conditions; even though they wore veils which, fortunately, were fashionable at the time, they were pathetically conspicuous. Treatment in all three cases was partly by X ray, and at one time when his machine for the work broke down he arranged to use another doctor's equipment temporarily. Rather than make three separate trips with them, he asked all three to come to his office on a certain day so they could go together, a walk of a few blocks.

It was like Father not to realize that a doctor escorting three veiled skin patients on a city street would attract attenion. They had hardly left the office when he saw his mistake. Men stared; a group of children scattered and ran; women held handkerchiefs over their noses and ducked in doorways or crossed the street to avoid meeting them. The four hurried on to their destination, but by mutual consent they left by different routes after their treatments and waited for the next one until Father's machine was repaired.

Alma Johnson was making good progress when for some reason the railroad company stopped issuing her pass, and she could not afford fare to the city. Father said he could give her the treatments at the Sloan office; his X-ray machine there was essentially the same except that it was operated by hand.

We no longer took patients in our home, so Father inquired around Sloan for a place where Alma could stay. He learned of a young housewife who wanted a girl to help care for her children in exchange for her room and board, and he went to see her. He carefully explained the circumstances and warned her of the girl's appearance; he assured her that Alma had been instructed in caring for herself so that there would be no danger of contagion to others. She agreed to take Alma; but when Father brought her, ready to stay, the woman took one look at her and covered her face with her hands. "Oh, I'm sorry," she said, "but I just couldn't have her here with my children."

Father was angry, but there was nothing he could do. And since another woman might react in the same way, it seemed useless to look further. He brought Alma back to our house, where the heartbroken child sobbed as she waited for the train home. Mother almost wept with her as she tried to console her. She didn't care to assume the responsibility of looking after a young girl, but it was unthinkable to let Alma stop treatments just when relief seemed assured, so she said, "I don't need another girl; when our two are home the house is full, and when they are gone there isn't much housework. But I think we should be able to find a place for you. Suppose you stay here for a few days and we'll look around." It took Mother only those few days to decide that she did need another girl if that girl was Alma.

Not only had the girl's Swedish parents taught her to work; she showed an inherent love for keeping busy and being helpful. When Mother went out to start dinner, she would find that Alma had already pared the potatoes and set the table. While we lingered at the table wishing there were not so many dishes, Alma would whisk them out to the kitchen and start to wash them. She answered the telephone before anyone else realized it was ringing. She was always ready to turn the handle on the X-ray machine for Father, and even Dr. Lacy sometimes called on her for help in the office.

She was a godsend for Mother, who no longer looked tired but now found time to relax; she had time too for piecing quilts and making rugs as she had always wanted to do.

When I worked on my trousseau I found Alma was an able seamstress. She even fitted my dresses; in her capable hands linens were quickly hemmed and laid away; then together we pieced a quilt. She never seemed to tire, but rather was so happy in doing things for others that she radiated an added warmth to our family circle.

Alma was with us for about a year, and at the end of that time her skin was clear except for a few stubborn spots on her nose. We were glad for her, particularly since after our big move we would have no place for her. A small apartment in the city would do for the folks, who would be alone most of the time.

Meanwhile plans were shaping up for Father, and he let it be known that he was leaving Sloan. Dr. Prescott had proven to be popular, sincere, and capable, and Father assured his patients that they would be in good hands. They reacted in various ways.

Most of the patients, realizing the change was inevitable, expressed themselves as pleased with the work of Dr. Prescott and wished Father well in the new venture. Others wept and implored him not to go.

One rawboned, sharp-featured woman burst into the office and demanded to know if it was true that Dr. Frear was deserting them. Father answered, "I'm sorry to say I find it necessary to leave my work in Sloan, Mrs. Beener. I'll miss good friends like you and Joe, but I'm not deserting you. I assure you that——"

"You'll assure me nothing," she said angrily, her face red, her eyes flashing. "Dr. Frear, I am telling you that you have neither moral nor legal right to go off and leave sick folks that depend on you for their very lives. When my Joe heard this morning that you're leaving he had to take to his bed. If he dies you could be held responsible."

"My dear Mrs. Beener," Father said quietly, "I've been very careful in choosing my successor. Dr. Prescott has had better training than ever I had, and he can take better care of Joe than I could."

"Better care? Oh, no, no! Oh, Doctor, you just don't know what you are doing to us." Her voice broke, and her anger spent, she left the office in tears.

Meanwhile Nels Solen, retired Norwegian farmer who had bought a house in the next block so that he and his wife could spend their remaining years near the good doctor, sold his house and moved to Sioux City.

Our house was put on the market. Not many people were interested in buying so large a place, but the Shannons, a farmer and his wife who wanted to retire to a comfortable home in Sloan, liked the house and found the price right. They were not in a hurry to take possession; we could take our time to move.

There was a mortgage of two thousand dollars against the property. It had been built free of debt but Father had borrowed on it to pay college expenses, first for Edna and me, then for Charley. The note would soon be due, but the sale would be consummated before that time, and the Shannons would pay enough in cash to more than cover the amount of the note. It could all be taken care of at one time: the mortgage satisfied, the deed transferred, and the balance of the money turned over to Father.

It could be, but Father found that it was not to be that easy. Unknown to Father, the man who had the mortgage planned to foreclose and was not easily put aside. He called at the bank and demanded that the note be paid before any other papers were made out, knowing full well that Father could not meet his demands.

On the morning of the day the transaction was to be closed, Father stopped at the bank to sign such papers as were necessary. Only then was he told that the note must be paid first. Sick and discouraged beyond any hope of meeting the terms, he went home to break the news to Mother, then left for his train to the city.

But in the employ of the noteholder was one of the boys Father had known as children in the Norwegian area. Young Olson was familiar with the deal, in fact he would have charge of the transaction at the bank. Evidently he remembered that this man who was in difficulty was the one at whose knee he had learned his first English and his letters as well. He remembered him too as the physician who had brought him and other members of the family through many an illness, and had shown for each of them a lifelong interest and sympathy in ways outside his professional calling.

Father had gone on the early train. I planned to take a later one to do some shopping in the city, and as I waited at the depot I saw Dr. Lacy coming up the walk. He never hurried, but now there seemed to be an urgency in the long, swinging stride. He was obviously pleased about something. "When you get to the city," he began when he reached me, "you'd better go right in and see your father. We have good news for him."

He went on to tell me that Olson had drawn two thousand dollars from his own savings account and had paid the mortgage against the house. There was nothing the holder could do but accept it. When the Shannons came in as previously arranged, Olson had gone ahead with the sale, and all was ready for Father's signature on some of the papers, and a check for three thousand dollars awaited him.

Glad to be the bearer of such good news I went directly from the train to the office. Father sat at his desk in the back room, his head buried in his arms. He looked up as I spoke to him, the picture of despair. I said, "Congratulations, Dad, your house has been sold."

"But it isn't sold," he said wearily, "the deal is all off."

"No, Dad, Lacy told me just before I left that the mortgage had been taken care of. He said——"

"I don't care what he said, Carrie. I was at the bank myself this morning. Now please just go away and leave me alone. You wouldn't understand. Nothing can be done and I don't want to talk about it." He turned back to his desk.

I hesitated; I wanted to tell him, but it would make matters worse to start an argument when he was in such a mood. He must have relented a little as he turned and saw me standing there helpless, for he said more gently, "Go on and do your shopping, then come back and we'll have lunch together." I seized the opportunity to divert his mind. Where would we eat? What time? Was this the day they served New England dinner at the Palace Cafe? Then I told him about a letter I had just received from Lon. As we talked he became more calm and I said, "Well, I'll go on to Martin's store, but first just listen to this." Before he could stop me I repeated the message from Dr. Lacy.

"But Olson couldn't do that," he protested. "He'd risk losing his money and probably get fired too."

"He trusts you, Dad. He knows you will pay him, and the check is right there to cover it. I don't know about his job. I hope he won't be fired, but he must have thought it was worth the risk."

"I don't believe a word of it," he said stubbornly. "But tell me again, just what did Lacy say?"

Presently I left him, moved almost to tears by the loyalty and generosity of his friend, ready to shout for joy that the business deal had been closed. He begged me to hurry back so we could talk things over. I made a few necessary purchases, then went back to spend the rest of the day with him. We would have all too few hours together from now on, and there was really little I needed for the simple wedding I had planned.

Lon's work would be finished early in October, and we had set October 12 as the day for the wedding. We were one of eight couples to be married that year whose romances had begun in Morningside College and most of whom had graduated, but Lon and I added an extra college touch to our wedding. The Reverend Mr. John Waterman who had graduated from Morningside in

June had just come to preach in our church in Sloan and we asked him to officiate. The *Sioux City Tribune* writing of the event used the headline:

MORNINGSIDE WEDDING FOR SURE!
EVEN THE PREACHER AN ALUMNUS!

I never considered having a church wedding; home weddings were then the rule, at least in Sloan. And I was glad that we were still living in the house Father built; it seemed so right to be married there. There was ample room for the twenty guests—relatives who lived close enough to attend, and a very few friends. Alice Lee, who was so like one of the family, came from eastern Iowa where she was teaching; her sister, Mary Ellen, and a high school friend, Anna Dubois, who was the great-granddaughter of the Indian chief, War Eagle, came to serve the refreshments.

Lon's mother had made my wedding dress of mousseline de soie trimmed with bias folds and soutache braid. I wore no veil, but pinned a rose in my hair, and carried a bouquet of pink rose-buds Lon had brought from a city florist. Mother had banked her prettiest plants and the chrysanthemums that were in bloom in the corner of the living room where we were to stand.

While Edna played the wedding march, I came down the stairway of which Father was so proud. Lon met me there, I took his arm, and we walked together into the living room for the short service. I remember Lon's firm "I will." I tried to make my vow equally convincing, but it sounded rather weak.

As we turned, man and wife, to face those who were so dear to us, I had a fleeting impression of Father's seriousness; of Mother in a pretty white blouse, her face turned away from me (but later I saw her wipe her eyes); of Edna sitting at the piano, as I always think of her; of Charley, quiet and aloof; and of Mother Hawkins, her lovely auburn hair like a halo in the soft light.

Aunt Mary in her black silk, her dark eyes twinkling, sat in the doorway to the dining room; beside her, quiet and dignified, sat Skipper, the big shepherd dog who had followed her from home. Just as the wedding march had started, Lon's four-year-old niece, Mildred Abbott, had slipped to the door and let Skipper in, and now she stood with her arm around his neck. My cousin, Susie Washburn, smiled as though she were happy for me; the mother of seven children, she was still a beautiful woman. Her brother, Ernest Smith, with tears in his eyes, appealed to Lon to "be good to this girl, my favorite cousin."

I remember mistily the congratulations and loving wishes, the refreshments, and the goodbyes that tried to be cheerful as we left for the train.

Lon had given up his plan for a trip to Niagara Falls so that we could spend a week in Pennsylvania with Aunt Cora and Uncle Dana. That too passed and at last we were in Washington, D.C., the exciting and glamorous city we were to call home for the next thirty-four years.

In about six weeks Father and Mother moved to Sioux City; soon after that Lon's family left to make their home in California, hoping that his mother's health would benefit from the warmer climate. So, for our parents as well as for us, the old way of life had ended, and we all would seek new friends and new activities in new places.

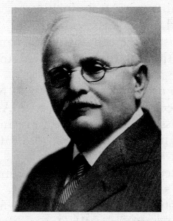

Dr. Frear as his grandchildren knew him. A mustache had reappeared, and the hair was white, but his step was buoyant as ever.

Chapter 16

GRANDFATHER FREAR

WHEN THE FOLKS learned that they were to be grand-parents they were pleased and excited. Right away they wrote me that I must come home for the event and let them take care of me. This seemed a good arrangement, for if I went with Lon for his season's work for the government, our home would probably be a room in a small hotel, a half hour's train ride from the nearest hospital; so we decided to accept their invitation. Lon planned to leave for Michigan in April, and in order to give him time to pack our household goods and put them in storage, I planned to go home in March. The baby was due in June.

Now Father had cared for many a mother-to-be and delivered many a baby. He had never lost a mother in childbirth, and the babies were almost without exception husky little animals. So in his letters he told me what a normal process it was to have a baby and urged me never to give a thought to my condition. Then as he thought things over he seemed to remember that this was *his* daughter and this would be *his* grandchild, and he must take every precaution; in the end he showed *his* lack of concern by going to Chicago to meet me.

After our arrival at home, to me he kept up a pretense of ignoring the coming event. I wasn't supposed to know that he called Mother from the office three or four times a day and kept a close check. No expectant mother ever got better care.

The big day was June 12, 1910, and about noon Stuart Frear Hawkins was born. He apparently met the approval of both grandparents. Father chuckled over the first lusty cry, admired the well-shaped head and broad back, and said under his breath, "By gosh, you are a dandy!" It wasn't long before I heard him at the telephone calling his friends and mine to announce, "This is Grandfather Frear."

Mother smiled as she dressed the little fellow and I could hear her whisper endearing names; from that hour she was Stuart's adoring slave. They both spoiled him, of course. The rascal demanded, and got, attention every minute of his waking day, which was a long one for he refused to sleep until he and everyone else were exhausted; still he was so lovable and responsive when played with that no one objected, least of all his grandmother. She loved to rock him and sing little Irish lullabies, and sometimes she would look up to smile and say, "He really is a good baby." I laughed to myself—I couldn't agree with her.

He had another devotee in his Aunt Edna, who taught piano at Morningside College and lived at home. When Stuart was six weeks old, Edna suggested that we take him to Sloan and show him to friends and relatives there. Father insisted that we come downtown early and stop at the office so he could introduce his grandson to his friends. That included office girls, doctors—everyone from the elevator boy to the officers of the trust company on the first floor, who owned the building. When the youngster had been exhibited and admired to his grandfather's satisfaction it was time to leave for the short walk to the station.

I started to pick up the baby but Father said, "Here, I'll take him. He's too heavy for you." Out on the street he settled his precious bundle on arms held straight out in front of him, reared back to get his balance and strutted ahead with his quick, short steps. His face beamed with pride and broadcast to all he met as plainly as though a sign were pinned to the blue bunny blanket, "My first grandchild."

Edna and I dropped behind with the suitcase, and we were amused at the expressions on the faces of people he met. A middle-aged woman nudged her companion, and both smiled so openly that Father turned and asked, "What's everyone laughing at? Ain't I holding him right?"

"You're doing fine," Edna answered quickly, "and we're almost there." He could not hear her aside to me, "They're not laughing at him. They're just enjoying the baby with him."

After a week in Sloan we returned to find both grandparents at the train to meet us, and Charley as well. He was home for the summer and when he thought no one was watching, added his bit in devotion to the first baby in the family since his own advent twenty-one years earlier.

Stuart grew and gained in weight, as well as in such social graces as were suited to his age. He showed occasional signs of indigestion but nothing serious and, since he was making good gains and was breast fed, Father said we should not experiment with medicines or foods. but leave him to the best doctor, Mother Nature.

When the baby was four months old, it was time to join Lon in the East. His work since May had been in New Jersey and was finished the first of October, when he went to Baltimore to continue work for his doctorate at Johns Hopkins University.

Both parents insisted that I write detailed reports of the baby's development—something that I enjoyed doing. Father was pleased with his physical progress for the first few months. But when the boy was weaned and should have had a variety of foods, none of them seemed to agree with him. Father was puzzled by this report, then became concerned when there was no further gain in weight and the boy became anemic. He and Mother carefully went over everything they had noticed while the baby was with them, and he blamed himself for not having discovered any possible congenital condition at that time. He talked with children's specialists; there apparently was nothing he could do at such a distance, but he would not give up, even though two doctors who saw the boy during this time were unable to diagnose the condition.

One of the men who saw him was Dr. Boston, a country doctor who worked with Stuart during the summer while we were with Aunt Cora in Pennsylvania. He seemed to be making some headway when we were obliged to leave for home. The other one, a prominent Baltimore physician, had dismissed the case when the boy was in a worse condition than when the doctor was called. I was afraid to have him come again.

So I continued to write to Father and ask questions. He never was too busy to answer in detail, and he discussed at length anything that worried me. He advised and suggested as best he could, also sent me the best book he could find on infant care, one more scientific than usually given to young mothers; he tried to fill in where the book left off. And always he said, "Now don't you worry. That boy isn't going to starve to death. Just keep on with the malted milk as long as it doesn't upset him, and eventually we'll find something else he can eat. Don't try to force him." Without Father's help I could easily have given up. At sixteen months Stuart weighed exactly what he had at four months— sixteen and a half pounds.

Patiently Father suggested one food after another to try, telling me what reactions to watch for and when to stop feeding it. Some were rather unorthodox, such as the thick piece of bacon, which he directed me to tie up "like an old-fashioned sugar-tit" for the boy to suck on. He chuckled over the report on that, for Stuart loved it. Here at last was some of the fat he needed badly, in a form he could digest.

Then, after inquiring among his colleagues, Father wrote about an outstanding pediatrician in Baltimore, where we were living. I called his office but was told that he took only cases sent him by other doctors. A few days later Stuart became very ill and I called again, and this time insisted on talking with Dr. Mitchell. According to him, Dr. L—— who had prescribed for Stuart a year before, in spite of the unfortunate results, was our doctor and should be called.

I said, "Dr. Mitchell, my Father is a doctor and I understand your position. But I know that even a good doctor sometimes makes mistakes. That doctor does not know what ails my baby, and after what happened, I am afraid to take a chance with him again. It would be a waste of time too—he wouldn't even remember us." I was crying now and didn't care if he knew it. "And I don't know anyone else to call. If you don't come, Stuart won't have any doctor, and he is a pretty sick baby."

"Mrs. Hawkins," the voice was very gentle now. "I will be there to see your baby sometime before noon."

He came within an hour. Except that he was younger, I saw

a strong resemblance to Father in his build and general appearance, his precise way of speaking, and even more in his sympathetic expression, his sensitive mouth, and kindly eyes.

After he had treated Stuart for this acute attack, Dr. Mitchell, as Father had hoped, diagnosed the condition that had been the cause of all our trouble. Reduced to simple terms, certain glands had been slow in developing. He explained further that it was such a rare condition he was not surprised that his friend, Dr. L——, had failed to recognize it.

After he had completed the examination and had given me careful instructions, Dr. Mitchell leaned back in his chair and studied me, much as I had seen Father do when he was particularly interested in a patient. Presently he said, "Mrs. Hawkins, what I can't understand is, how have you kept this boy alive? Not one baby in a hundred survives this condition, even with professional care, and you seem to have brought him through alone."

"But I really didn't do it alone, Dr. Mitchell," I said. I told him about Father, and how faithful and painstaking he had been in working with me—answering questions, advising and encouraging me. The doctor listened carefully and asked many questions, then said, "You are very fortunate to have such a father. It would require rare understanding of medicine, and endless work and patience as well, to cover all phases of such a case by correspondence, as he has done. And you have been wise to follow his instructions and not give up as you might so easily have done." He paused to look at Stuart, who had fallen asleep.

"Now I will be happy to help you with the boy," he said, "and I can assure you that, having come this far, if you will keep on with your good work, you will have less trouble from now on. And I feel safe in promising you that by the time Stuart is four years old he will have overcome this idiosyncrasy and will be a strong, healthy boy."

His prognosis proved correct; we soon had the boy on a nourishing diet and had little trouble thereafter, and none at all after he was four. When Father saw him again, on our visit home when Stuart was five, he marveled at the boy's physique and wanted me to tell him everything about the treatment and the diet he had been given. He shrugged off any credit for his part in bringing Stuart through the trying months of infancy, but I could see that he felt well repaid for the time and work he had devoted to the problem. He looked over the sturdy little chap with the bright eyes and red cheeks, felt his muscles and strong back, looked down his throat, and said to Mother, "Well, Sue, I guess he'll do. All he needs now is to get filled up with some of our home-grown vegetables."

Mother turned to smile at her grandson as she set dishes of creamed peas and baby beets on the table. "We'll start on that right away," she said. "Dinner is ready."

At dinner Stuart endeared himself anew to her when he asked, "Grandma, may I have another slice of that delicious bread?" for she was proud of her baking. And when, on taking his third piece of chicken, he said, "Chicken is my best food, Grandma. Let's always have it," she agreed at once. She stuck to her bargain too, for a time. But one day Stuart went to the refrigerator for a snack and found there was no chicken. He evidently decided to do something about it.

Mother heard loud squawking out in the chicken yard and ran out the back door, and just in time. Stuart had asked a neighbor boy, Burdette Kindig, to help him, and as Mother reached them, Burdette was holding her old setting hen on the chopping block while Stuart tried to balance the heavy ax to strike. From that time on, Stuart's diet included a greater variety of meats; that, of course, was no punishment, for Mother was an excellent cook.

She was now fifty-six and, while she was a little overweight, her posture was good and she was still attractive. It proved to be our last visit with her, and Stuart, who of course could not remember our earlier stay with her, was always to think of her as she was now, with her gray hair curling softly about her face and neck, her ready smile and warm tender eyes reflecting the love she felt for her family and friends. She had kept young by taking an interest in young people. They now lived a block from Morningside College and she kept her spare rooms filled with boys from the college, making sure that they were properly mothered while in her home.

Then further to enrich her life there came another grandchild, little Martha Alice Schuyler. Shortly after I left for the East with the baby in 1910, Edna had been married to Will Schuyler, a young druggist in business at Danbury, about fifty miles from Sioux City. When they had first started keeping company, Father used to try, without much success, to tease them about their first date when Edna was a mere infant and Will was a mature one-year-old.

"You both went to Ladies' Aid with your mammas," he told them. "There was one didy satchel for the two of you; in it was a bottle of milk for Edna in case she cried—one of those old flat bottles with a long tube fastened to the nipple—but Willie found it and did away with it. But he furnished the transportation. He had one of those fancy reed baby carriages with a fringed red parasol to keep the sun off. Edna just snuggled down beside Willie and both went to sleep." Now, about thirty years later, their blue-eyed girl with curls like her grandmother's rode in the 1915 model, a folding go-cart.

Six years after our visit to Iowa, Stuart and I went to meet Father at his old home in Pennsylvania, now the home of his brother, Dana, and wife, Cora. Father tried in vain to keep up with his eleven-year-old grandson, who wandered about in the woods and fished in the mountain streams he himself had loved as a boy. It was too fast a pace for the sixty-seven-year-old man, and soon he was obliged to give it up. However, in order to have a part in the adventure, he offered to pay the boy five dollars for the first trout he caught. One fish after another had been brought for his inspection but none had filled the requirements when Father left for a week to attend a medical convention in Boston. On his return, Stuart could hardly wait to tell him, "Grandpa, I think I caught a trout while you were away. Wait till I show you." He ran up the hill to a big rock and returned with a desiccated fish which had lost all resemblance to any particular species.

"This apparently is, or was, a fish," Father said, as he examined it as well as he could and still keep it some distance from his nose, "but how am I to know it is a trout?"

Uncle Dana was appealed to. "Well, as I remember it," he said, "I'd say it looked something like a trout when he caught it," and there was a twinkle in his eye.

"It was shaped like a trout," Aunt Cora said, "and it had scales and fins and everything, and I particularly remember a very troutlike expression in its eyes." She too was laughing.

Father doubted that it was good policy to pay anything on such questionable evidence, until he learned how hard the boy had worked to have something to show him. After catching the fish, Stuart had put it in the spring near the house and faithfully dug worms and caught flies to feed it, but his fish died in spite of all he could do. Keeping it to show his grandfather then presented a problem. Finally he had carried it up to this rock and kept watch to see that none of Aunt Cora's nine cats or any other animal carried it off. Father wanted to be fair, so they compromised and he paid the boy a bounty of two dollars and a half.

"And now here's another way for you to earn some money," Father said. He handed Stuart a clipping which he took from his wallet and said, "If you will memorize this poem, I'll give you five dollars. And what's more, if you will live by its principles, you will lead a happy and successful life."

The poem, called "Work," written by Angela Morgan, had been published in *Outlook*. It extolled those old-fashioned virtues after which Father had patterned his life. It was a good poem and it would seem to deserve wider publicity than, apparently, it had. It began:

> Work!
> Thank God for the might of it,
> The ardor, the urge, the delight of it—
> Work that springs from the heart's desire
> Setting the soul and the brain on fire—

There were forty-one lines—quite an assignment for a small boy on vacation in Pennsylvania's wooded hills, but Stuart persevered and was able to collect his reward; and now, fifty years later, he can repeat most of the poem.

Father came home with us to Falls Church, Virginia, across the Potomac from Washington, and we continued our visit. Father and Stuart did some sightseeing together, including a trip to Mt. Vernon. After a tour of the buildings there, they spent a quiet hour sitting on the lush green lawn, while Father held forth with reminiscences and homilies. Next morning he discovered his anatomy had acquired a bright scarlet belt with matching ankle-trim. It was his first experience with "chiggers." He tried all the remedies we had to offer for the severe itching caused by the tiny red larvae, but they offered little relief. Then he wrote a prescription and sent Stuart to the drugstore. The result was a lotion that took care of the nuisance in a most effective manner, a remedy that was in great demand as long as we lived in Virginia.

Chiggers notwithstanding, Father enjoyed Virginia, but his dedication to his work was strong. He soon returned to Iowa. There was an added attraction at Edna's now, for by this time she had four interesting, lively children, who looked ahead eagerly to the frequent visits of their grandfather.

When Martha reached age ten she was given the poem "Work" to learn, as Stuart had done, to earn her five dollars. But she had what she considered an even better source of income. Martha had protruding front teeth, something that her grandfather felt reflected on his professional standing; he said such a disfigurement could not be tolerated in a doctor's family, and he promised Martha that when the dentist decided it was time, he would pay her a dollar for every month she had to wear braces.

Considering financial gains above her discomfort, Martha relished her good fortune. The day arrived when she met her grandfather at the train, the wide grin displaying a metal band on her teeth, and hailed him with, "Hey, Grandpa, I've got a big joke on you. The dentist says I've got to wear these things four years. Know what that's going to cost you? Forty-eight dollars!"

On my next visit to Iowa, I spent more time at Edna's than I had on previous visits, for now we had a small daughter, Barbara Sue, who enjoyed being with her cousins. But Stuart was fourteen, old enough to be companionable with his grandfather, so he spent most of his time in Sioux City. Mornings they walked together to the office and the boy had a chance to glean from the old man's experience and philosophy bits of wisdom that made a lasting impression; they exchanged ideas on all sorts of subjects—one generation with another.

At one time Stuart asked him why he did not get a car to save time in getting to his patients. Father pointed out that now most of his patients came to him at the office. Then he went on to say that speed was not always desirable, and he spoke of the tendency of ambulance service to emphasize speed to the neglect of other important factors. He thought the modern automotive ambulances went much faster than was necessary, that there seldom was an emergency where the time saved made up for the confusion and the resultant bad effect on the patient. He felt that the tendency was for medical decisions to be forced under too high pressure and that not enough time was taken to consider the patient. "Possibly that sounds like the opinion of an old country doctor who is opposed to progress, in this case the stepped-up procedure of modern surgery," he said apologetically.

"It makes sense to me anyway," Stuart answered. During their talks, he asked so many questions about headaches and their significance and causes, that Father became suspicious. When he learned the boy was subject to headaches he started him on a series of medical examinations with the best specialists in the city checking every possible cause for the trouble. He was found to need glasses and they were provided.

Often instead of going out at noon they prepared lunch in the office, probably bacon and eggs, and Stuart was amused when, after the dishes were washed, Father rinsed them with a weak solution of hydrochloric acid. Father laughed when he saw Stuart watching. "Now I know they're clean," he said, "and sanitary."

At first Father couldn't share his grandson's enthusiasm for baseball. He had attended a game twenty years ago, he said, and vowed he would never see another. He considered it a waste of time and money. But he was all sympathy when he realized the boy worried about the World Series being played at the time. So he inquired around until he found out that the game would be shown, play-by-play, on a scoreboard posted on a certain street corner, the 1924 equivalent of televised baseball.

With the excuse that the boy might become lost, he took Stuart to the corner, then waited, chuckling over his excitement. Then while Stuart explained the plays, the game itself took hold of his grandfather. He stayed until it was over, and when the Washington Senators had won the World Series, he was almost as happy as Stuart. On returning to the office he was reminded that he had missed two appointments, but he confided to me later, "That was more fun than I've had since I can remember. Those two patients will probably come back, but if they don't—well, doggone it, it was **worth it.**"

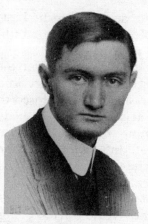

Soon after this photo was made, Charles Frear, now Dr. Frear, left his father's office for World War I service in France.

Chapter 17

A SON, TO BECOME A DOCTOR

GOING BACK several years to the fall of 1914, we find Charley, at twenty-five, within two years of finishing medical school—only somewhere in the classroom or dormitory his name had lost the diminutive form and he became "Charles" as intended, though many of his close associates and, of all people, his mother, still used the nickname he had as a little tike, "Stub."

To Lon and me he was Charles; and when we learned that he planned to attend an eastern school and so have an entire change of scene, we asked him to make his home with us. We could help him cut down expenses and would see that he had wholesome food and care if he became ill. This pleased the folks on all counts. Mother would not worry about her boy if he were with us.

Father had always been able to visit Charles at school; he had kept in touch with his teachers and followed the progress he made in various courses. It is doubtful if that ever encouraged the boy to study harder—probably not. Just what was expected of us in that regard, Lon and I were not sure, but we resolved that our responsibility would end with giving Charles a home. We considered him an adult, and as such capable of running his own life. If he studied, that would be fine. If he spent his evenings out, where he went and with whom were his own affair.

Of course we were pleased when he showed real interest in his studies. He had registered at Georgetown University, and soon after school opened he started bringing home with him a young Filipino, good looking and always well dressed. Night after night they studied together. Through the wall that separated his room from mine I sometimes heard their voices. Charles would explain at length some phase of their assignment, then ask, "Do you get that, Vic?"

The first try seldom was successful, and Charles would say, "All right, Vic, look at it this way!" and start another approach. Again, later, "Well, let's go back to the beginning of the chapter and start over." After several trials apparently Vic would understand, and they would proceed to another topic.

I admired Charles' patience with a poor student, and one day I said, "I hope Vic appreciates all the help you are giving him."

"But it's the other way around, Sis," he said, laughing. "Vic helps me. He is slow to get a point, partly because of the difference in language and background, but once he gets it he never forgets. I get things quickly, but have a poor memory. However, by the time I've explained something from a half a dozen angles and got it across to him, I've got it so I retain it; so it's a perfect setup for the two of us."

Occasionally Vic ate with us, and Charles sometimes brought other students and friends for dinner—maybe a shy, homesick nurse or some girl he had discovered from Iowa. They were always the sort of young people we could like and enjoy.

And we had no reason to wonder about his evenings out after the first Friday evening he was with us. He came downstairs dressed for the street and Lon asked casually, "Are you going out among them?"

"Yeah, in the interest of a broader education," he said with a one-sided grin. "It seems to be a necessary part of student life to go to this theatre once a week." He mentioned a playhouse known for risqué vaudeville. "I want to be sure I'm not missing anything."

About nine thirty he came in. Lon looked surprised. "I thought you were going to a show," he said.

"I was, and I did," he said and added dryly, "The show was supposed to be rotten, and it sure was, so I got up and left." He made no further comment then or later, but he didn't go again, to our knowledge.

Certainly Charles needed no suggestions from us in conducting either his social or his school life. On the financial side the picture was different. It took some restraint for us not to interfere in some of his extravagance. Like Father, he had a casual disregard for the value of money, and he had had no training in using it wisely.

Probably because Father recognized the trait in himself, he was too lenient with the boy. He was over-generous when he had the money, although at other times necessarily close. He wanted his son to have an easier time than had been his; he had worked for every cent he ever possessed.

Of course Charles worked too; even as a little chap he was always ready to take a job to earn money, but knowing that his father could be counted on for all necessities, he spent it on whatever at the moment pleased his fancy, so that he had never established a pattern of saving. And now, too far away for Father to keep in touch with his money problems, Charles would be on his own for two years.

He left for Washington in time to stop off for two weeks in Pennsylvania. Aunt Cora took a great liking to him, and believing that the boy would spend wisely if he had money available without writing to Father for every dollar he needed, she decided to finance his first term in Washington in her own way; she gave him a check that, carefully handled, should have covered his expenses for that period. Now for the first time Charles had a bank account.

After paying his tuition and buying textbooks, his next check was for two expensive suits of clothes. A dinner jacket followed. Then Lon and I were amazed when a desk and chair, bookcases and a rug were delivered. They were from a secondhand store and were good values; but we had naively thought the room was already furnished. In less than a month Charles' money was gone. Father hustled around and sent more and wrote that he felt well paid when Charles' first report came and he had excellent grades.

As I look back now, I believe it was about this time that

Charles began to show a deep interest in the study of medicine. It had not always been so. There was a time in his teens when, although he had no real objection to becoming a doctor, he wanted to look around. For a time he considered other vocations, but without much enthusiasm for any one of them; Father expressed a willingness to be satisfied and to help with any course the boy wanted to follow, but Charles felt it was only a gesture. In the end, having no definite plan of his own to offer, he went ahead with the plan laid out for him, but he resented, unfairly perhaps, that the choice had been Father's instead of his own.

There came a time when his resentment boiled over. It was after his year with us, and before his last year at Georgetown University. I was home for the summer, and on this evening dinner was over and the four of us were in the living room, Mother and I with our mending, Father with his newspaper, and Charles stretched out on the davenport.

As usual, the conversation drifted to Charles' plans for the coming year. Lon and I had been able to cut expenses for him during the past year and would have been glad to have him with us again. However, we planned to move and would live farther from Georgetown, possibly thirty minutes by streetcar. Understandably, Charles wanted to live near the school and with other students. And in order to do that, he said he must have money on deposit where he could get at it and not have to write home, then wait, for what he needed.

Father laid his paper aside and said, "But that is out of the question, Son. Your room and board will cost so much more, and to advance it and start a bank account—well, you know that I can't send money, only as it comes in; you know too how that is in small, scattered amounts. I'm not complaining, but my dear boy, you must realize what a strain it is to keep you in school. I've had my nose to the grindstone ever since you started."

"All right, but I'm not exactly to blame for that. It's what you wanted me to do. Why in heck did you get me into this if you couldn't afford it?" Charles sat up and faced his father. "You knew medicine is about the most expensive course a man could take. It costs more, takes longer, and the work is so darned hard that a fellow can't take any time out to earn anything on the side."

Father was too stunned to answer. Never had he seen Charles in such a mood—not that he lost his temper; rather, he calmly gave expression to feelings that too long had smoldered within him. Now he asked, "Why didn't you send me to business school? Or agricultural college? A plain college education might have made it possible for me to teach, or maybe become an athletic coach. Or if college cost too much, I'd have made a good carpenter, and enjoyed it, too."

Mother and I had kept silent, rather than make matters worse, but now, evidently in the hope that she could divert the trend of the argument, she said, "Or an undertaker. That might have been a lot of fun."

Charles turned to her with a half-smile. "It might at that," he said.

But Father, pacing the floor, now seemed determined to defend himself. "You never wanted to do anything else," he said.

"How do you know? How could I know? I never heard anything from the day I was born except that I was going to be a doctor."

Father stopped in front of him and said stubbornly, "You know very well I've always told you to do as you please. I've said I'd help you in whatever you wanted to do if you didn't want to be a doctor."

Charles laughed dryly. "And in the very next breath you'd talk about plans for medical school. I knew very well that I wasn't supposed to do anything else, so I went along with it, but all the time I've felt like a puking pup without guts enough to do anything on my own. For years I swallowed my pride and any thought of what I might like to do."

He paused, then went on more calmly. "I know now that I wanted to be a doctor all along. Medicine fascinates me. In fact. I love it. And after all these years I know that I never could have chosen anything but medicine. But why on earth wasn't I allowed to make the choice for myself?"

Mother could stand it no longer. Her voice unsteady, she said, "We don't have to decide on plans for fall just yet. Why don't we let it go for tonight? It's bedtime."

Father looked at her as though he might protest; then, shoulders drooping, he turned and went into his bedroom. Charles buried his face in his hands and was silent for a while, then he got up and said, "I'm sorry, Mother. I guess I said too much," and he, too, left for bed.

There seemed little we could do, but Mother and I discussed the situation for some time before we went to bed. One thing was certain, Charles must be made to see how unreasonable his demands for a bank account were, considering the way he had gone through the one he had had the previous fall.

The next day I went down to the office and found Father looking so dejected I could have wept for him. He spoke at once about Charles' outburst. "I can see now that all my life has been wrong," he said. "I have failed at every turn. I never realized before what I was doing to my boy. I have pushed him—made it impossible for him to take any other course—and now it's too late to make amends. I don't see how I could have been so blind."

"Don't blame yourself, Dad," I said. "Charles was absolutely unfair. It was a vicious attack and I know how it must have hurt you. But I believe there is another side to this. It seems to me Charles is just waking up to himself, just beginning to realize he hasn't taken the responsibility he should. Now he's looking for some place to put the blame. After he thinks things through I believe he'll come out all right."

"But the fact remains that he's absolutely right about it," he said. "I've made a mess of things."

"Not by a long way," I said. "You've probably made some mistakes—all parents do—but on the whole you have followed the best course possible for Charles. A more rugged boy could have tried a lot of things, earned money to finance wildcat schemes, found himself by trial and error, and then come back to the study of medicine." He was listening hopefully. "With Charles it was different. His life had to be directed. Thanks to the good care you and Mother have given him, he is in good health now; but if he had been left to his own devices, it might have been a different story."

He walked over to his desk and sat down, and motioned me to a chair. After a bit he began to talk, more hopefully now, about finances. "I'm a poor manager, but maybe if I planned more carefully I could ease the money problem," he said. "I must confess, I never had given a lot of thought to the boy's side of it. I only thought of myself. It is hard for him to spend wisely when money comes in so irregularly. And it is embarrassing for him, too. I've got to do some thinking on this."

Meanwhile Mother and Charles had talked things over and she was able to show him that he had failed to prove either his right to having a lump sum given him for expenses, or his ability to handle it. He was ashamed of his outbreak and apologized to

Father. Eventually the two men found a more realistic approach to the money problem; Charles returned to Washington and a room with classmates near the school, but with a firm resolve to be more fair and consistent in the use of money.

Back at Georgetown he became even more interested in his work. Moreover, he confided to Lon that he could see now that he was far ahead because his course had been directed even when he was too young or too unsettled in his thinking to plan for himself; there had been no scattering or waste of time or energy, and now he was grateful for all the planning that for a time he had so thoroughly resented.

Eventually it was over, and after graduation in 1916, Charles was home. Father's worry, the financial strain, his sacrifices, were a thing of the past, his dream of having a doctor-son realized. Charles seemed as happy to work beside Father and profit by his experience as Father was to have him. There wasn't a large practice to share; Father did some general work, largely for former patients who came up from Sloan or who had moved to the city; he made medical examinations for several insurance companies; and he continued his special practice in diseases of the skin. But the office, the equipment and library, and the backing of an established physician, things that were usually big items for the newly-graduated doctor, were waiting for Charles and gave him a splendid opportunity to start in and build up his own practice.

Father was very proud as he introduced his son to his friends and patients. Charles was nearly six feet tall, slender, with deep-set eyes, high forehead and firm chin, and he had a quiet, reserved manner that gave him a professional air. Unlike Father, he was careful of his appearance; he talked little, still he never seemed at a loss to carry his share of the conversation, and his dry wit often eased the tension and made strangers feel at home with him. As he became acquainted he soon had patients of his own, and nothing made Father more proud than to have someone come in and ask for "young Frear."

Mornings they left together for the office and returned in the evening to share the day's experience with Mother at the dinner table. Then Father usually buried himself in his newspaper, and for Charles the evening belonged to Mother. For her he had an unusual devotion. During his childhood it had been necessary for her to watch over him closely, and while she certainly did not

170

neglect her two daughters, it was always "little Charley" who needed her most and was closest to her. However, her devotion had been wisely administered and she had not made him dependent on her; he was not a "mamma's boy" and he was unselfish and thoughtful toward her.

The rapport between them seemed to be a stabilizing influence on the young man, for he gave them little cause for worry except during illness. He and Mother became very close as they tried to make up for all they had missed while he was away at school. When Mother did the kitchen work or cleaned house, Charles was right there with her, helping her more, so she told us, than either of us girls had ever done. And as he worked he talked over his plans and dreams and confided in her about his girl friends.

Then, too, Charles had a rare understanding of Mother's problems and her desires that we girls, and even Father, lacked. He was sensitive to her craving for good music, art, and lectures on world travel and social problems. There were cultural advantages in the college town that she had missed in Sloan during the struggle to educate us children and to meet the demands of a country practice, so Charles took her often to events on the campus.

On the other hand, Mother was able to interpret for him some of Father's moods and shortcomings; she encouraged him to be patient with the old-fashioned ideas and to wait for the time when they could modernize the office and extend their facilities. Through her he gained a deeper appreciation of Father's fine character, and she instilled into the young man some of her own loyalty and devotion. It was a profitable and happy year for the three of them.

Within the year, World War I had started and doctors were needed in the service. Charles' experience in the practice of medicine was only beginning, and he would have liked to stay with Father a while longer. But he was young, single, and in good physical condition, and had had some training in the National Guard; under the circumstances there seemed only one thing for him to do, so he enlisted. He was sent first to Medical Officers' Training Camp at Fort Riley, Kansas. By autumn he was stationed at Camp Cody in New Mexico as Assistant Sanitary Inspector of the 34th Division with the rank of lieutenant. Inspection of camps and training of other men for the work held him there, and he was not sent overseas until the war was nearly over. He did not see service at the front; however, after the war ended, he spent about seven months as captain in charge of the 76th Sanitary Squad at Beaux Desert Hospital Center near Bordeaux, France.

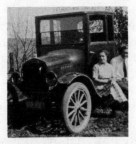

The age of the horse and buggy doctor was over. The postwar years belonged to the auto, and to Dr. Charley and his bride.

Chapter 18

ADJUSTMENT

WHEN THE ARMISTICE was signed, Charles was one of the many boys in France who counted the days until they could come home—while thousands of the loved ones who waited for them in America were stricken with the epidemic of flu that raged in this country. No one who lived through those days will forget the horrible experiences of the fall and winter of 1918. In Washington many government workers who were away from home for the first time fell ill and were dead before they were missed by their fellow workers or their landladies. Young parents were taken suddenly and their small children left without food or care until discovered by neighbors. Little was known about treatment. Hospitals were overflowing; the shortage of nurses was acute.

In Sioux City also the epidemic was severe. Mother was taken ill suddenly on Thanksgiving Day, then developed pneumonia. No nurse could be found for her, but six of Father's colleagues dropped in to help in whatever way they could. Aunt Mary came up from Sloan. Edna, leaving her two little ones with her husband and a neighbor, joined her. They wired me, but both Stuart and I were just recovering from the flu, and war priorities made it impossible to get train reservations.

Everything possible was done for Mother, but in spite of the loving care, she grew steadily worse. On December 6, Father, standing by, helpless and heartbroken, saw a change in her condition and said, "Sue, are you going to leave me?"

She smiled up at him . . . and she was gone.

Before Charles left home for the service, the folks had built a home in East Morningside. They had written me how comfortable they were, and how happy. They had all modern conveniences, still they had room for chickens and even for two pigs; together they had raised a big garden, and together had canned fruits, vegetables, and meat. At the time of Mother's death, Father's brother, Dana, was with them, and now he tried to help by doing the work while Father was at the office.

Father wrote that Dana was a good housekeeper but not so good at planning meals. He didn't know how to prepare fresh vegetables nor even the canned goods there waiting to be used; he couldn't dress a chicken; so they lived largely on oatmeal, potatoes, bread and butter, and honey. Father, who was fond of meat and needed fruit and vegetables in his diet, added in his letter, "but tonight I cleaned some celery for breakfast."

He wanted to keep the home for Charles, who was nearly thirty, and who had looked forward to having a home as soon as he could settle down. He wrote from France that he had worked hard on his French and apparently had a flair for it, since he was often taken for a Frenchman; he had also been invited to some Bordeaux homes. He mentioned one girl, Germaine Martin, but indicated no special interest in her. But Father knew that, even if Charles remained single for a while, he would appreciate a home.

However, before long, Uncle Dana left for the East and Father was alone. For a time he tried to find a young couple or a woman to keep house for him, but one letter he received rather discouraged any further effort to find a housekeeper.

A widow who had learned of the circumstances wrote that she was sure they could work things out to the advantage of all concerned. She could come at once, she said. Her daughter who was to be confined in June would come in May so that she could have her mother's care, and Father could deliver the baby. She understood that I was coming home for a visit and she said that it would be best for me to be there when the baby arrived so I could take over the housework and she would be able to devote all her time to her daughter. Since Father would of course make no charge for delivering the baby, she would make a reasonable price and come for ninety dollars a month! And that was in 1919, when a dollar was worth one hundred cents! But Father felt that the "all-one-happy-family" arrangement would be a poor bargain at any price.

Meanwhile he had a letter from "Nick," his younger brother who had lived with us during the nineties and for a time had practiced dentistry. He had married, as his second wife, a young woman with a Pennsylvania Dutch background. Assured that "Minnie" was a good housekeeper and cook, Father sent for them. Now he had some of his own family with him and he was more contented.

Then in June, Charles was finally separated from the service and came home. He brought with him his French bride, the former Germaine Martin, a pretty girl with flashing, dark eyes. Germaine was from a well-to-do family and had extravagant tastes and the idea, held by so many French brides, that American men had "plenty, plenty monee." I could see something of the many-sided problems she and Charles had to face when they stopped to see us on their way to Iowa. After we searched the Washington stores and failed to find the kind of shoes she wanted, she said, in French, "It is all right. If I can't find them in Sioux City, I'll run in to New York sometime and get them."

In Germaine's immediate acceptance of "Mon Papa Frère," one could see a reflection of Charles' affection for Father. He pretended to be indifferent to her outspoken devotion; however, we could see that he was pleased with her attentions—even with her impulsive kisses.

Unfortunately, her affection did not extend to all members of the family. Two good women with more different ideas could hardly be found than Germaine and Minnie, and neither was happy in the presence of the other. Their personalities and activities served only to keep them farther apart. Germaine spent the mornings in her room, where she polished and shaped her fingernails, put just the right touch of mascara on her long lashes, and applied makeup that enhanced, never cheapened, her natural coloring. In a more practical mood she might make a bewitching beret from a scrap of velvet, or a scarf from a wisp of chif-

175

fon. She wanted to sparkle for "Mon Charlee and Papa Frère"—
and sparkle she did.

But her winning ways did not impress Minnie who, neat in
her crisp print dress with her hair smoothed back, spent the
morning preparing vegetables carefully so as not to waste them;
she baked bread, canned fruit, and did the laundry, being especially careful with Father's shirts; she did all those things which
made the home comfortable, and still kept down expenses. But
Germaine was not impressed with Minnie's efficiency—she wasted
a good opportunity to learn the practical ways of an American
woman's life.

Understandably enough, she wanted to get away and have a
home of her own. Charles, too, became restless. He was not interested in diseases of the skin and felt he needed to get more experience in general practice, so he decided to go to Salix, where
Father had started, and build a place for himself. Father tried to
hide his disappointment, hoping that Charles would eventually
come back to work with him.

Then Nick and Minnie grew homesick and left for the East,
and Father was alone again. Train service to Salix was good, and
he often went down for the night, partly because he felt they needed him. Charles had many night calls and Germaine was timid
when left alone. Besides, she was not an experienced cook in any
language, and since she could not read English, the labels and instructions on cans and packages and recipes in cookbooks were of
no use to her, so Father supervised the cooking and did much of
the housework, too.

I laughed when Father wrote me about his "visits" there; he
went on to say: "Both Charles and Germaine want me to stay
with them permanently. I appreciate their offer, but I still feel my
calling is in the field of materia medica rather than in the kitchen.
Also, I think I would rest better if I didn't know everything about
Charles' work. He certainly has plenty of it to do, and is pleasing
people, too, but I worry when there is no need for it. I think two
years of this will satisfy him and he will be back in the office
with me."

But at the end of that time, Charles moved to Holly Springs,
the quiet hamlet nestled in the hills about six miles east, where
they built a home and appeared to look forward to a permanent
location.

Now there seemed to be no further reason to keep a home for

Charles, so Father sold the house in East Morningside. "My friends urge me to marry again," he wrote to me, "but your mother spoiled me for any such move. She was so interested in my work and assisted and advised me in every way, and, as I realize now, steered me away from many a wild dream. No other woman could mean anything to me now. I would constantly measure her against Sue and find her wanting. Some friends argue that by marrying again I would do a kindness to some good woman needing a home. Even if that were so, I do not care to be so generous."

Had he cared to take advantage of it, Father would have been welcomed in the home of any one of his children. In fact, Edna and Will investigated the possibility of selling their Danbury drugstore and going into business in Sioux City in order to make a home for him there, but it did not seem feasible, and Father would not consider leaving his practice to go to Danbury and live with them. And he was determined not to drift into something less than a solution to his problem of adjustment, but to face the situation squarely. He knew that, for the present at least, neither his practice nor his home life would include Charles.

Undecided about living quarters, he slept for a time on a comfortable couch in the office and got his breakfast on a gas plate. Then, on the insistence of his friends that it was not safe to sleep in the building alone, he took a room far enough uptown that walking to the office gave him the exercise he needed.

Meanwhile he looked around to see where he could be of service. His very aloneness gave him a point of contact and sympathy with others. Girls employed in the building came to him with their problems and found him an understanding listener, and medical advice was given them without charge. High school girls and boys from the college all found in him a friend. Deaconesses, Catholic nuns, and the Salvation Army brought him charity cases, many with problems he could help adjust.

Evenings were long and he began to widen his interests. He joined a nature study club and the Sioux City Academy of Science and Letters. He met with six other men interested in the history of the area and they started a Pioneer Club that soon became a large, active organization. He wrote papers for the programs of some of the meetings, and many of them were published. He also wrote on temperance and the use of tobacco, projects he had long had in mind. One pamphlet, "The Perniciousness of the Cigarette," was widely distributed by the W.C.T.U. Always interested in national and family history, he took out membership in the Sons of the American Revolution.

Father had written me of his various activities, and on our visit in 1924 I enjoyed hearing more about them. After six years, he still missed Mother keenly, but he lived a full, contented life. Besides his writing, his organizations, and new friends, he had close touch with his children by correspondence, telephone, and frequent visits. Charles and Germaine drove up often from Holly Springs.

Father and I and the children, Stuart and Barbara Sue, went down there one day; Edna with her family drove up from Danbury and we all had dinner together. Germaine had become a good cook, and the dinner, which included some of their home-grown vegetables with fried chicken and mashed potatoes, had a definitely American flavor, especially the dessert, which was ice cream; Germaine gave this dish her own special touch when she served generous portions and set them at our places before she called us to dinner.

Charles and Germaine seemed to be happy and well adjusted, and a feeling of mutual respect and affection was apparent between Charles and Father. Stuart stayed for a visit with his Uncle Charles, while Barbara Sue and I went back to the city with Father. There were a few days remaining before the children and I would leave for California where Lon was to be stationed for a year.

I spent the afternoons at the office, and while the little girl took her nap in the back room, Father and I would visit. One day I suddenly realized that he heard me perfectly when I spoke in an ordinary tone of voice. I asked him, "What have you done about your hearing? It seems to be all right."

"My hearing hasn't improved," he answered, "but I have taught myself to listen. I forget myself and concentrate on the other person and what he wants to tell me, and I have very little trouble." I thought it a very practical application of his usual consideration for others. It added to the enjoyment and to the privacy of our visit.

On my last afternoon with him we had put Barbara Sue down for her nap. Father lingered for a long look at this littlest grandchild, who had the soft curls, arched brows, and slightly turned-up nose, as well as the name, of his beloved Sue; then he joined me in the consultation room but stood looking out the window. It was cold for October, and a heavy wind dashed rain against the pane. There would be few interruptions this afternoon. I spoke of Charles. "He seems to be doing well in Holly Springs. Do you think he will be ready to leave there and come in with you before long?"

He turned then and said, without the slightest sign of resentment, "I don't think Charles will ever practice with me again."

"But that isn't right after all you've done for him—you've worked for it and planned on it for so long!" I said, surprised at his apparent acceptance of the fact.

He sat down and settled himself in his swivel chair before replying. "Well, I'll admit that I was disappointed when I first realized it, but now I see that was a selfish way to look at it, and I am really proud of him for making the choice he has."

"What are his plans?"

"I think I told you that Charles is interested in psychiatry," he said. "At first I tried to discourage it, but he has convinced me that it is the right field for him." He leaned back in his chair, hands spread with fingertips touching, watching me closely as he talked. "And when we were there this week, he told me that he is going to look for a place in an institution where he can work into special psychiatric practice, and at the same time take advanced work in some school."

"But why psychiatry? There is so little interest in it."

"That's just the point. Psychiatry is in many ways the least advanced of all the medical sciences, and there is a very definite need for it. Why, would you believe—?" He stopped and shuffled through some papers on his desk. "Well, I had some statistics, but never mind. Anyway, more than one out of every three hundred people is in a mental institution—not to mention borderline cases and even advanced ones who should be there; and they don't get the care they should have. Attendants who look after them are chosen largely for their brute strength. In some institutions they still have patients in chains; some wear handcuffs or straitjackets, and a great many are strapped to hard beds."

"Why don't they do something about it?" I asked lamely as I began to realize the seriousness of the situation.

"Because they don't have enough trained people to do the work. That is their biggest problem." He went on to say that psychiatrists were now beginning to realize that a large percentage of cases were curable, and that even more were preventable, with

179

proper care and understanding. "That is the field Charles hopes to work into—prevention of insanity." His eyes lighted up. "Do you know, Carrie, that's a real opportunity for service! To help people to live happy, well-adjusted lives!"

"With your enthusiasm you might even consider taking it up yourself," I said, smiling at him.

"I might if I were younger," he said, nodding his head; "I might at that. The humane side of it appeals to me. And at least the boy has a better reason for his choice of a specialty than I had for mine." He laughed as he remembered. "When the Sioux City College of Medicine was organized, no one wanted to teach dermatology. They finally prevailed on me to give it a try, and as I developed the course skin cases started coming in." He paused. "But Charles has chosen because of the conviction of a need, and a sense of responsibility toward that need."

I couldn't forget the years Father had worked and looked forward to having Charles as an associate. Furthermore, I realized that if Charles went into institutional work, Father would be alone in the city; he should have one of his children with him. "It still doesn't look right to me," I said.

"Look at it this way, my dear girl," he said earnestly, throwing out his hands in emphasis. "In planning for Charles, I have had a goal all these years—something to work for—and that was good for me and for all of us. Obviously, thirty years ago I couldn't have had the vision, the foresight, to plan for my boy to be a psychiatrist. That was a field I had heard little about. But this is a different age, and Charles has been around, and has a broader outlook than I had. He has discovered something to which he considers it worthwhile to devote his life."

"In telling you, did he seem to realize what a disappointment it would be to you?"

He thought about that a bit. "Well, probably not. I think the big plans he has in mind overshadowed everything else. And since I have thought it over, I'm proud that he knew he could depend on me to see things his way. For him to have given it up for fear of hurting me—that would have been tragedy. And now, even though I could not see the Master Plan, I am glad to have been used for its fulfillment. Perhaps this is to be my one contribution to humanity—to raise a son for such a worthwhile cause."

I couldn't answer that; I could only think of the struggle he must have had to reach such complete acceptance of Charles' plans, and the time he probably spent in prayer. I watched him as he got up and looked around the room. One wall was lined with bookcases, for he had a fair library; his equipment for treating patients was adequate; but the furniture was old and worn, the curtains lifeless, the rug threadbare. Then he faced me and said, "I shouldn't try to run another's life. I haven't done too well myself. After forty years of practice I should have an up-to-date office, full of patients, and at least enough money to keep me from financial worry."

"You have enough patients if you would charge them enough," I told him. "If you had many more you'd be hustling from one to the next one and wouldn't have time to listen to their real problems. Then you'd miss the chance to really help them, and that's what you live for, mainly." I laughed and added, "And if you had money, you'd just give it to someone else who needed it."

He chuckled. "Maybe you're right." He came back and sat down, the chair squeaking under his weight. "Well, as a matter of fact, I never did covet wealth for myself. But I always hoped I'd be able to leave a legacy for my children, even if only a small one. I wanted to make life easier for them than it was for me. It seems to me that I have failed my children."

"You? Failed your children?" I cried. "Why, Dad, you gave each of us a good education, after earning every cent of yours all alone. You've already made it far easier for us than it ever was for you. And as for a legacy . . . well, Dad, there's something I've been wanting to tell you." I paused—we Frears did not express our emotions easily. "You know, people from all over the country come to Washington, and I travel about a little too. Quite often, I meet someone from Sioux City, or even from Sloan. I've been away quite a while and usually they don't know me, so I say, 'You might have known my father, Dr. Frear.' I'm always proud to speak of you. I never need to hesitate for fear they know you unfavorably."

He studied his fingernails and did not look up as I continued. "And if they know you, or of you, their reaction is always the same. They say, 'Oh yes! Dr. Frear is the one who was so good to me . . .' or to a son, or to a friend. And then they tell me of something you did, sometimes as their physician, more often beyond the demands of your profession, to help someone in trouble. Many times they will say, 'Dr. Frear is the kindest man

181

I ever knew.' " Now with misty eyes he watched me as though trying to be sure I told the truth. Then I said, "Do you know, Dad, you couldn't leave me a better legacy, and I just wanted to tell you that I am humbly grateful."

He tried to answer me, then gave it up, plainly embarrassed by the turn the conversation had taken. Just then Barbara Sue appeared in the doorway and ran to his outstretched arms. He held her close and buried his face in her dress. Then Charles and Germaine came bringing Stuart, and we all went out for dinner; there was no time for further intimate conversation.

I was glad we had had our little visit, for when I told him goodbye at the station that night, I bade farewell to Father as I had known him and loved him ever since I could remember.

O the snow, the beautiful snow,
Filling the sky and the earth below.
Over the house-tops, over the street,
Over the heads of the people you meet. . . .

—JOHN WHITTAKER WATSON, *Beautiful Snow*

Chapter 19

AND ONE CLEAR CALL

ALL WAS QUIET in the west wing of St. Vincent's Hospital, except for the pounding of the steam radiators as the heating plant struggled against the intense cold and furious wind of an old-fashioned blizzard. It had started snowing just as I stepped from the train in Sioux City a few days before. Although I had spent the last twenty years in the milder climate of Washington, D.C., I still recognized the fine, dry snow that filled the air, coming from all directions at once, as the forerunner of some real Iowa weather.

Father seemed warm enough, I thought, as I fluffed up his pillows and massaged the leg and arm that a week before had suddenly become useless. There was little for me to do, but he needed someone with him constantly, so they had sent for me. I slept in his room uptown, and spent my days at the hospital, relieving his special nurse while she went for meals or to rest.

Charles had come for a few days, but he had recently taken a position as house physician at a mental institution in Mt. Pleasant, Iowa, so the time he could spend with Father was now limited. Edna and Will still lived at Danbury, fifty miles away, with their five lively children, the youngest only a few weeks old. Barbara Sue, now four years old, who had come with me, was with Edna and enjoying herself there, but I missed her.

The nurse had admitted very few people to see Father. This

was not to my liking, for I enjoyed talking with callers, many of them family friends whom I had not seen for years. Often I would go out in the hall to speak to someone the nurse was about to turn away, but as a rule she did not give me time. There was, for instance, the old man who had appeared at the door, dirty, unshaved, and shabby. She was very abrupt with him, but before she closed the door in his face I had caught his look of blank bewilderment. I stepped out in the hall hoping to see him, but he had disappeared.

On inquiry I learned that he was someone Father had known as a boy in Pennsylvania, homeless now, his mind failing. They said he had been to the office several times in the past week, and couldn't understand why the doctor wasn't there to take him out to dinner as he had done so many times.

At another time the nurse looked down the hall with evident disapproval, and I said, "I'll take care of this one." Going to the door I saw, as she had, a short, plump man wearing clothes much too long for him; his overcoat, sweater, coat, and vest all were unbuttoned and swung out behind him as he swaggered down the hall with both hands in his trousers pockets, peering about through thick lenses for the room number. When he told me his name, I remembered him as one of the boys who had roomed with the folks at one time. Now he edited a paper in a small town about forty miles away.

There were no words of sympathy or vague offers of help if we needed him. This man went straight to the point. "I have a heated car and good tires," he said, "and I will be glad to take you down to Edna's to see your little girl, now, or any time you want to go, and bring you back whenever you are ready." With a newspaperman's instinct, he had learned that Barbara Sue was with Edna. His offer would have meant for him to drive a hundred miles in the storm had I been able to accept, and I was very grateful, but I could not leave Father.

His next suggestion was a very practical one. "As you probably know," he said, "I worked in banks and sold insurance while I was here in college, so I have contacts and know my way around." He might have added that he also knew what a poor manager Father had always been, but he tactfully avoided that. "I wondered if I couldn't save you and Edna some work if I find out for you what insurance the doctor has, and where and what his bank connections are."

I hadn't had time even to think about that problem, and a complicated one it was. Gratefully, I accepted his offer. He returned in about two hours with a typed list of many items, including among others an insurance policy with a loan against it; the details of the lease of Father's office, which, of course, must be given up and the furniture and equipment disposed of; he told of an off-and-on checking account in one bank where he also had a safe deposit box which only Edna could open. His errand accomplished, he left, still without any expression of sentiment or sympathy, but I was deeply moved. And the nurse would have turned him away!

Edna came up the next day, planning to look into Father's business. She was relieved to find so much had been done for her. "It would have taken me days to ferret all that out," she said. "I hardly knew where to start." She paused as two women came to the door. A determined looking, elderly woman, round shouldered, her head bundled in a heavy shawl, was followed by a modernly dressed, younger woman, who apologized at once. They were from out of town, she said, adding, "Mamma insisted on coming. This foot has bothered her for weeks, but she refused to see anyone but Dr. Frear. When he wasn't in the office, nothing would do but I must bring her over here."

The older woman added her bit: "Ven I have this on other heel—five year it been—nobody know vat iss. Nobody care much. Nobody help me but Dr. Frear. I come back." She had already unbuckled her old style overshoe, removed that and the wool sock underneath. The gray cotton stocking came slower—it stuck to her heel.

Fortunately the nurse was at lunch. I looked cautiously down the hall, then stood holding the door closed.

Father had been drowsy and uninterested all morning, but here was a patient! Instantly he became the professional man, alert, efficient. "All right, Mrs. Weiger," he said, "tell me about your heel. Let's take a look at it." She put her foot on the chair by the bed. He tried to raise up, then looked at us helplessly. He couldn't reach her foot with his good hand; he couldn't even see it.

In a flash the old lady climbed up to stand on the chair and put her foot on the bed beside him. Edna turned and lifted him a little, so he could both see and reach it. There was an ugly running sore on her heel. He probed around it gently, asked a few questions, and said, "I see what it is—same as you had before. That medicine helped?" He asked for a prescription blank. We gave him pen and paper, but then he was frustrated again. He couldn't write. But Edna, being familiar with prescriptions, was able to write down what he dictated.

The patient meanwhile had re-dressed her foot and got her purse from the pocket of her dress. "Never mind that now," he said. "Let me know how you get along and I'll send you a bill later." Both women thanked him profusely and left.

"Well, that was quick work. Good thing no visitors came," Edna said as she washed his hand. "Or nurses!" she added, and we laughed. Father smiled weakly, but he was tired. He sighed, closed his eyes, and soon was asleep. The nurse returned, and I left with Edna to go to the bank.

The next morning when I came the nurse told me Father had had a bad night, and she had been up with him. Now she was leaving me in charge for the day, so she could get some rest. She gave me a meaningful look and closed the door firmly, after putting up a NO VISITORS sign.

She had said he would probably be no trouble for he would sleep all day. But instead, he was restless, and even the soft foot-steps on the rubber-covered corridor floor disturbed him.

I tried not to distract him, and was standing at the window watching pedestrians battle the wind, and cars plunge uncertainly into drifts when Father called me to him.

"Tell me, Carrie, is there a NO VISITORS sign on the door?" he asked.

I hesitated. A good nurse would never admit a thing like that. But I wasn't a nurse. I was only the patient's daughter, and he had taught me to tell the truth. "Yes, Dad, there is. The nurse put one up. She wants it quiet so you can get some sleep."

"You go take it down," he begged.

"I can't go over the nurse's head," I argued weakly.

"Now listen, girl, I am a doctor, and I know what's good for me and what isn't," he said earnestly. "Every time I hear footsteps I think someone is coming to see me and they can't get in. If any-one braves this storm to call on a sick person he should be ad-mitted. It worries me so I can't sleep."

That was so like him; I knew he spoke the truth, and after all, I was not bound by hospital rules, so I said, "Dad, if I take that sign down, will you promise to go right to sleep, and not talk much if anyone comes in?"

"I won't need to talk at all," he insisted. "They'd rather talk to you anyway, and I'll probably sleep right through. I really am tired." He paused, watching me, and when I still hesitated, he coaxed, "That's a good girl; you take it down, and leave the door open a little so they'll see you. Then they'll come in, and you can tell me all about your visit later."

I removed the sign and soon he was asleep. He was right—people did want to talk to me, but not in the way he thought. They wanted to talk about him, to tell me of something he had done for them, always with his rare gift of sympathetic understanding: maybe just an encouraging word; but often at a sacrifice on his part, he had given help needed in facing some crisis in life.

The first visitor to come was a slender girl with a sweet face, yet self-effacing and serious for one so young. She slipped in quietly as I nodded to her. "Father is asleep—" I began.

"It's all right," she said. "I'll not wake him, but I wanted to come in and see him."

I started to give her my chair, but she indicated one beside the bed. "Do you mind if I sit here? I'll be very quiet. I just—I just want to—to be near him for a little while." Her eyes pleaded for understanding. I assured her it was quite all right. She seemed inclined not to talk—to be absorbed in her own thoughts—so I turned back to the book I had been reading.

But after a few minutes when I looked up and smiled at her as I turned a page, she said simply, "I am Elsie." The name meant nothing to me.

I explained, "I think my sister would know you, but I live in the East and don't know many of Father's friends. Were you a patient of his? Or maybe you worked for him?"

"I was a patient first. . . . Later he got me a job in the building. Oh, I can't tell you all he did for me. . . . I'm going away soon, and I don't know what I'll do when I can't see him any more." She choked back a sob.

"Surely you'll be back," I said.

She shook her head. "Not a chance. There won't be money enough. I'm taking my grandmother down to my aunt in Missouri. She's going to give her a home. The fare will take all we can scrape up. I'll have to get work and stay there." She looked at

Father through her tears. "I can't bear to tell him. . . . I'll wait, and I'll come in every day 'til I go."

Father stirred a little. What if he should wake up and not recognize this girl, to whom it meant so much just to be near him? But I needn't have worried. He looked up just then and saw her. "Why Elsie, child!" His voice was very gentle. "You shouldn't have come out in this storm to see me." There was real affection in his voice as they talked for a few minutes, then she slipped out as quietly as she had come.

Edna filled in Elsie's story for me. Raised in an environment that provided very few of a girl's needs, physically or spiritually, she had come to Father for medical advice at the suggestion of a deaconess. Father learned that she had quit school a few months short of graduation, and he insisted on knowing why. He did not scoff at her embarrassed answer, but encouraged her to talk. Later he checked with the deaconess and with the school matron, and learned that Elsie had told the truth: she really lacked clothes to make a respectable appearance at school.

He asked her to make an estimate of how much she would need to finish high school. She named a moderate amount that would cover everything from badly needed underwear to a graduation dress. He hadn't money to give her, but he took her to a department store and vouched for her, agreeing to pay her bill if she failed to do so.

Elsie was graduated with honors, her creative writing having attracted special notice. Father got her a job, part time until school was over, then full time, and she had met the bills for her clothes as they came due. Then she saved her money carefully, hoping in some way to get more schooling, but that money now was to be used to take her away.

After Elsie left, visitors continued to come in spite of the storm—people from all walks of life. Children came, and old men; a Unitarian minister, although Father was a Presbyterian; a poet whom Father had encouraged and who was now getting recognition; two high school girls who apologized to me for not coming sooner—Aunt Lottie had died, they said, and they had waited until they could get themselves in hand, because if the doctor found out about it he would feel so bad.

A five-year-old with his parents, from a farm near Sloan, came to tell Father about his new pony. This one was a girl pony, he

188

said, "and she'll grow up to be a mamma pony and have a baby pony, and I'm going to give it to you."

A judge who knew just the right things to say made a brief call, followed by a middle-aged man in a sheepskin-lined coat and felt boots, whose drooping sandy mustache, blue eyes, and ruddy complexion marked him as a Norwegian farmer. He stood reverently by the bed for a few moments, then wiped his eyes on his sleeve and left without saying a word.

A doctor from out of town, whom Father had helped to get started on his medical career twenty years earlier, stopped in as he brought a patient to the hospital. Accustomed though he was to seeing illness, he broke down and cried as he left the room.

Soon after the nurse returned, Sister Placida beckoned to me from the hall. She had dropped in occasionally during the day to see if I needed assistance. Now she took me to an unoccupied room and said, "You will not be disturbed. Lie down and rest." She patted me affectionately on the shoulder, "And have yourself a good cry." I needed no urging.

By the end of the week we had given up the nurse, who was badly needed for a surgical case, and I spent full time at the hospital, sleeping on a cot in Father's room.

On Sunday a young teacher came from a town about twenty miles north. Father was asleep, and I said, as I often did to visitors, "He may not recognize you when he first wakes up."

The young man spoke up quickly, "Oh, he wouldn't know me anyway. I'm just . . . well, I'm just one of the boys he has helped. He never saw me but once."

Of course I looked surprised. "It was this way," he continued. "It was the beginning of the spring term, and I was to graduate from Morningside in June. I had paid my tuition, had my books, and waited on tables for dinner and supper. But doing the best I could, I couldn't raise money for room rent. Dr. Frear heard about it and sent me the key to his office, and I slept there on his couch until I graduated."

"What about breakfast?" I asked.

"I usually didn't have time—had to leave for early classes about seven. But sometimes I'd fix something on his gas plate." He laughed. "He had 'help yourself' signs on all his supplies. And since I was only there nights, I never saw the doctor till I returned the key. Then he wouldn't let me thank him—said he hadn't done anything—but without his help I'd have had to quit school. He might not even remember; he has helped so many. But I saw in the paper that he was in the hospital, so I just ran down to see him on my day off."

Toward evening the storm abated for a time, and a young couple drove from their home thirty miles over in Nebraska, bringing with them their three-year-old boy, named Frear for Father. They said they wanted the boy to see the good doctor who had befriended the mother when she was a stenographer in another office. They were sure that seeing Dr. Frear would make him a better man, even though he was too young to remember. The little chap showed an interest in the visit that suggested that its importance had been impressed upon him beforehand.

It was on one of the coldest days of all that the visitor came who stands out foremost in my memory. I knew at once that he was a farmer of the more prosperous kind: a farmer as the Iowan knows him, with a dignity, a sense of humor, and a philosophy of life that comes from working close to the soil. When he told me his name, Lige Adams, I remembered him and his farm in the foothills east of Sloan. I had been in his home in my childhood and had taught school not far from there later.

Father was asleep, but Mr. Adams and I visited for a while, and I was glad for news of friends over in the hills. I thought of his twenty-mile drive, for it was bitter cold, even though he had a heated car and there was now a good road. I said, "It was a long way for you to come to see Father on such a day as this, Mr. Adams."

At first he did not answer, but sat looking at Father for so long that I wondered if he had heard me; then he began to speak, slowly, quietly, as though each word was weighted with memories.

"Forty years ago next month your father came to see us . . . at night, in a worse storm than this. . . . I remember the date because it was the night our son was born. . . . The prairie was a solid blanket of snow; the roads, even the fence-posts were completely covered. . . . There wasn't a landmark that could be seen in such a storm, even in daylight. . . . I never did learn how he found his way, but he found it. If he hadn't"—his voice dropped almost to a whisper—"I would have lost my wife and baby. . . . It wasn't very far for me to come."

He was still looking at Father but I felt that he was seeing, instead, a young wife who suffered in agony while he stood by helpless, hearing again the doctor's cheerful "Hullo" as he drove

190

up to the door, remembering the welcome cry of a new-born infant.

"Forty years ago next month," he had said, and it occurred to me that the night he had told about was just a few weeks before I was born. What a night that must have been for Mother, knowing the danger her husband faced. Then, little by little, the story I had heard years ago came back to me, of Father's ride across the prairie in a raging blizzard. And, remembering, I could picture my mother as she paced the floor in her lonely vigil throughout the night, while her whispered prayer—"Father! O Father! Bring him back to me!"—reached up above the snow-laden wind to Him whose hand could guide the way through the blinding storm.

Father's last summons came on a cold March morning, just before daybreak, as many another call had come to the old country doctor. We were saddened by his passing, yet we knew he was glad to go; for often during the long months of his illness we had heard him pray, "Take me home! O Father, take me home!" And we shared his faith that he would find Mother waiting for him. We seemed almost to hear him calling: "Sue? Oh, Sue! I've come home!"